V&R unipress

Interdisziplinäre Verortungen
der Angewandten Linguistik

Band 23

Herausgegeben von

Sylwia Adamczak-Krysztofowicz, Silvia Bonacchi,
Przemysław Gębal, Jarosław Krajka, Łukasz Kumięga
und Hadrian Lankiewicz

Die Bände dieser Reihe sind peer-reviewed.

Silvia Bonacchi / Małgorzata Godlewska /
Łukasz Kumięga (eds.)

Anti-Vax Discourse in the Context of COVID-19

Local Perspectives with Global Implications

With 7 figures

V&R unipress

MIX
Papier aus verantwortungsvollen Quellen
FSC www.fsc.org FSC® C083411

Bibliografische Information der Deutschen Nationalbibliothek
Die Deutsche Nationalbibliothek verzeichnet diese Publikation in der Deutschen Nationalbibliografie; detaillierte bibliografische Daten sind im Internet über https://dnb.de abrufbar.

Gedruckt mit freundlicher Unterstützung der Universität Gdańsk und der Universität Warschau.

Gutachter: Prof. Waldemar Czachur (Universität Warschau)

Umschlagabbildung: © Silvia Bonacchi
Druck und Bindung: CPI books GmbH, Birkstraße 10, D-25917 Leck
Printed in the EU.

Vandenhoeck & Ruprecht Verlage | www.vandenhoeck-ruprecht-verlage.com

ISSN 2749-0211 (print) | ISSN 2749-022X (digital)
ISBN 978-3-8471-1881-7 (print)
ISBN 978-3-8470-1881-0 (digital) | ISBN 978-3-7370-1881-4 (eLibrary)

Contents

Local Perspectives

Łukasz Kumięga / Małgorzata Godlewska / Silvia Bonacchi

From COVID-19 Discourses to Anti-Vax Discourse: Contexts, Social and Socio-Scientific Positioning, and the Reversal of Epistemic (B)orders

Abstract

This contribution aims to focus on the medical, psychological and social aspects of anti-vaccination discourse in the context of COVID-19 with a twofold purpose: the first is to reconstruct some fundamental aspects at the macro- and micro-discursive levels; the second is to provide impulses for a critical reflection that (de)constructs the epistemic (dis)orders that characterise the analysed area, in order to subject them to scientifically based reflection. At the same time, some meta-discursive considerations are presented regarding the question of discourse analysis as a tool for action on social reality.

Keywords: COVID-19, vaccine conflict, text in context, discourse studies, psyche, medicine, society, globality, locality.

The following volume invites us to consider the COVID-19 pandemic from the perspective of its discursive constructions in the context of anti-vax movements. This approach assumes a dialectical relationship between local dimensions and global implications, which is illustrated through American, German and Italian anti-vax discourses on COVID-19 and its various manifestations.

In doing so, it departs from the entanglement of these discourses with medical, psychological and social issues, which seem to determine their specificity at a microdiscursive level, especially in media and professional spaces. These discourses are argued to be part of the existing and widespread debate on the rationale of fighting contagious diseases with the help of vaccines.

With its potential to eradicate dangerous diseases and decrease mortality, vaccination safety is one of the great visions of the modern era. At the same time, it is not merely directed to individual health and illness, but it may control collective health conditions. Preventive vaccination programs always aim to

Łukasz Kumięga, University of Gdańsk, ORCID: 0000-0002-8034-3593.
Małgorzata Godlewska, University of Gdańsk, ORCID: 0000-0002-3425-4899.
Silvia Bonacchi, University of Warsaw, ORCID: 0000-0003-3914-1233.

optimise the "social body" or "public health", ensuring a feeling of social security via trust which is nourished by the "dream of immunity" (Thießen, 2017, 9; Colgrove, 2006), a concept by which Foucault explains social power (Foucault, 2004, 25). Becoming a real "device of prevention" ("Dispositiv der Vorbeugung", see Bröckling 2012), immunisation makes the social body resistant to dangers and threats. Since the beginning of the 19th century, in the fight against smallpox, diphtheria and polio, against tuberculosis, measles and influenza, societies negotiated ideas about humanity and models of society, conceptions of scientific progress and security (Thießen, 2017, 30–37) in alternating phases of trust, scepticism and criticism. The debate about vaccinations shows persisting continuities and breaks in risk perception and in security concepts.

This complex process reemerged in all its strength and was charged with new tensions and polarisations by the outbreak of the COVID-19 pandemic, which shattered the promising vision of immunity due to the very high death toll recorded in all parts of the world. The dispute about the necessity of vaccination reared its head again: Should the state be allowed to enforce the inoculation of individuals in the interest of the general public? A strongly polarised debate with an extremely high potential for conflict followed the forced administration of the vaccine, which ultimately led to the end of the pandemic by 5 March 2023, when the WHO officially declared the COVID-19 pandemic emergency over.

At this point, it is worth recalling the key events of the pandemic, which began in Wuhan, China, in November 2019. It then quickly spread to all continents, becoming a worldwide epidemic with the uncontrollable onset of the virus causing a severe acute respiratory system infection labelled SARS-Cov-2.

The COVID-19 was the third outbreak in the first two decades of the 21st century caused by an animal coronavirus transmitted to humans, following the Severe Respiratory Syndrome (SARS) in 2002 and the Middle East Severe Respiratory Syndrome (MERS) in 2012 (Coronaviridae Study Group of the Inter national Committee on Taxonomy of Viruses, 2020, 1). In contrast to the first two outbreaks, which did not expand to become global pandemics despite their high fatality rates – 9.5% and 34.4% respectively (Pustake, Tambolkar, Giri & Gandhi, 2022, 10), the new wave of contagion was recognised, after an initial moment of disorientation, as a life-threatening disease that spreads worldwide at immense speed with an estimated average fatality rate of 3% (Wang, Horby, Hayden & Gaoet, 2020, 471). According to Worldometer, a regularly updated coronavirus monitoring system in place from January 2020 until 2024 (when countries stopped recording and providing statistical data on the pandemic), the total number of COVID-19 infection cases in Europe amounted to 253,406,198, including 2,101,824 deaths. Thus, COVID-19 turned out to be a global pandemic with strong local implications, a fact that became fully apparent with the introduction of restrictions on the freedom of citizens and the production of vaccines by multinational pharmaceutical companies starting in March 2021. During the pandemic, discrete anti-coronavirus restrictions were imposed upon social communities in every country affected by COVID-19, including travel limitations, quarantine, wearing protective masks, and national or regional lockdowns. These preventive measures were heterogeneous in every country and related to their governments' anti-COVID policies. The urgency to create a vaccine for the COVID-19 emergency led to compressed research cycles that significantly shortened the standard vaccine development timeline, in some cases reducing clinical trial phases over a period of a few months or weeks, a process typically conducted sequentially over the course of several years.

Let us briefly consider the particularities of the emergence of the pandemic in the countries in question, namely Italy, Germany and the USA. At the beginning of the pandemic, between January and May 2020, Italy became the centre of the outbreak with the highest infection rates. Despite a well-functioning health care system and competent epidemic preparedness, the country reported 31,500 cases of infection and 2,400 deaths due to COVID-19 in the first four weeks of the pandemic (Chow, 2020). The total number of COVID-19 infection cases in Italy reached 26,723,249 while the number of deaths rose to 196,487. Thus, Italy was the first country in Europe to face the brunt of the pandemic and implement a lockdown, banning all social gatherings and public events, and closing schools and businesses to minimise the risk of coronavirus transmission. The Italian government adopted diverse measures for the pandemic waves with their peaks in April and November 2020. The earliest decision was to introduce a lockdown related to northern towns most severely affected by the virus, before imposing the national lockdown on March 11, 2020 (Paterlini, 2020). In the first wave, national restrictions involved a ban on travel between regions, locking down all schools and universities and almost all businesses with just a few exceptions. Furthermore, Italy was the first country to initiate relaxation of these anti-COVID-19 measures in the sense of a regionalisation in the second November–February wave of the pandemic in 2021 (Merkaj & Santolini, 2022, 287). The security measures were subordinate to the coronavirus risk assessment in a particular region. For this reason, the country was divided into three zones where anti-COVID-19 measures were evaluated and introduced varyingly: the red zone signified a high risk of infection and strict measures, the orange zone – a moderate risk, and the yellow one – a low risk and the least strict measures (Merkaj & Santolini, 2022, 288). Although the anti-COVID-19 policy was determined by the government for the whole country, decisions concerning territorial needs and specific anti-COVID-19 procedures were discussed together with regional representatives in roundtables and introduced locally thereafter (Merkaj & Santolini, 2022, 287–288). In May 2020 a gradual relaxation policy was implemented which encompassed permission to travel between regions without justification, and the reopening of selected categories of businesses such as museums, restaurants, churches and sports facilities, albeit with the use of protective equipment and respect for social distancing rules. Due to an increase in coronavirus cases in the autumn of 2020, the government returned to more rigid anti-COVID-19 measures, adopted after the evaluation of the risk of the virus spreading in the country's regions. With the introduction of a complex prioritisation mechanism (medical personnel, vulnerable categories, socially exposed categories), Italy was the first country to start the vaccination campaign. After the official authorization by the EMA in March 2021, compulsory vaccination and the "Green Pass" (the EU digital certificate of vaccination) were introduced in Italy. In spring 2021 anti-vax protests started all over the country. The preferred arenas were the mass media, urban spaces (squares, streets, vaccination centres, see della Porta & Lavizzari 2022) and digital platforms. Social media, in particular, became a space of aggregation and conflict during the pandemic (see Bonacchi's contribution in this volume).

In Germany, the first cases of COVID-19 were identified in Munich, Bavaria, in January 2020 while the first two deaths caused by the coronavirus were announced in March in Essen and Heinsberg, together with alarming information about a 20% increase in COVID infections across the whole country (Inverardi & Nienaber, 2020). Overall, during the pandemic, Germany recorded 38,828,995 COVID-19 infections and a resulting 183,027 deaths. In Germany, the anti-COVID policy included social distancing, wearing protective masks and national lockdowns, though without the zone-based policy. From March 2020, after the detection of new infections in Essen and Heinsberg, schools as well as universities were locked, nursing homes were isolated from visitors, fitness clubs, restaurants and cinemas were closed, national events were banned, people were forced to work from home while supermarkets could stay open only on the condition that they introduced protective masks (Bosen & Thurau, 2021). The country's borders with Austria, Luxembourg, Denmark, France and Switzerland were closed except to goods and commuters (BBC, 2020). It is worth noting that Germany closed its borders as the last country in the region, regardless of early decisions to isolate imposed in Poland and the Czech Republic, and despite the WHO labelling Europe as "the epicentre" of the coronavirus (BBC, 2020). After the end of the first coronavirus wave, the German government launched a smartphone application, Corona-Warn-App, to track and alert anyone who had come into contact with people who tested positive for COVID-19 (Bosen & Thurau, 2021). In November 2022, with the escalation of COVID-19 infections, new anti-coronavirus restrictions were announced: apart from a curfew in Berlin, catering, hotel and tourism-related businesses ceased activities and social gatherings were limited to 10 people. Finally, anti-COVID-19 compulsory vaccinations and the European Green-Pass were introduced, though with a delay in contrast to other countries, for example the UK (Bosen & Thurau, 2021). The lockdown, as well as a national vaccination rollout, resulted in the significant containment of the coronavirus which allowed Angela Merkel, at the head of the German government, to rescind in April 2020 the national lockdown and slowly ease other anti-COVID restrictions across the whole country. In January 2021, a new national lockdown was imposed due to an increase in infections and the alarming number of deaths – 80,000 by April. Despite a subsequent temporary decline in infections, the fourth wave of the coronavirus swept through Germany despite the national vaccination plan. In December 2021, the new government enforced obligatory anti-COVID-19 vaccinations for health workers, a decision deemed controversial by some (Bosen & Thurau, 2021). The debate between supporters and critics of vaccination measures quickly spread to all social arenas (Plümper, Neumayer & Pfaff, 2021).

Apart from Europe, North America also suffered excessively due to the outbreak which, just in the USA, led to 111,820,082 COVID-19 infections and 1,219,487 deaths following the disease (Worldometers.com). According to Johns Hopkins University's mortality analysis, which calculated the number of deaths per 100,000 citizens in each of the twenty countries most affected by COVID worldwide, the mortality ratio was 1.1% in the USA, 0.7% in Italy and 0.4% in Germany, placing these three countries in the middle of the list of the evaluated countries (Johns Hopkins University Coronavirus Resource Center). In the USA, regulations concerning anti-COVID-19 measures highely depended on local governments and their policies, and varied in terms of the terminology of the implemented protective policy. The first decision to introduce "containment", specifically a ban on individuals' movement from home, was announced on 12 March 2020 in New Rochelle, New York. Nevertheless, the restriction did not involve the individuals' movement but the closure of schools and a ban on large social gatherings, including religious ones (Jacobsen & Jacobsen, 2020). Within a few days, other American counties were forced to impose similar restrictions on travel and social gatherings, though under a different and relatively misleading term, "shelter-in-place". This phrase was associated in the Californian states with a warning to "stay-where-you-are" announced during natural disasters such as wildfires (Jacobsen & Jacobsen, 2020), which did not convey a sense of lockdown or curfew, nor did it the limit individuals' movement or social life and business activities. Subsequently, the terms "shelter-in-place" as well as "lockdown" and "safer-at-home" were used interchangeably by state officials, thus frequently leading to confusion (Jacobsen & Jacobsen, 2020). The first decision to officially restrict citizens' movement was announced on March 19 in California, later in New York, and subsequently in six other states: Connecticut, Louisiana, Ohio, Oregon, Washington, and West Virginia (Jacobsen & Jacobsen, 2020).

It is noteworthy that the anti-COVID-19 policy in the USA differed during the presidencies of each of its two leaders to oversee the response, Donald Trump and Joe Biden. In the first phase of the pandemic, Donald Trump's administration did not announce any federal anti-COVID-19 restrictions. What is more, the president's controversial views on how to fight the coronavirus using non-scientific and ill-informed methods, such as injections with cleansing products or irradiation with UV light (BBC, 2020), were frequently cited as contributing to individuals' distrust towards the U.S. government's anti-coronavirus policy and for misinformation about COVID-19. The first rigid anti-COVID-19 measures imposed nationally in February 2020 were related to travel restrictions regarding those arriving from China and subsequently involved the government's recommendations to refrain from traveling to other countries. Anti-coronavirus guidelines, "15 Days to Slow the Spread", were announced by the U.S. president on March 16 with recommendations for social distancing and avoiding social gatherings in large groups. This relaxed attitude towards the pandemic was criticised by researchers and state officials who expected more rigorous federal measures to prevent the spread of the disease (Sheikh, 2020).

Stricter anti-coronavirus regulations were mandated nationally with the start of Joe Biden's presidency and the introduction of 12 official orders for the whole country during the first weeks of his administration, and stipulated, amongst other measures, wearing protective masks and officials socially distancing in federal buildings (Bradner, Klein & Hickey, 2021). Biden's administration prepared orders to be enforced nationally, which included obligatory vaccinations for officials and medical care, but the concept met with partial opposition. This divergence in the attitude towards the pandemic manifested by each of these American presidents can be rationalised through the politicians' contrasting political and social views and their dissimilar media self-representations constructed through disease narratives. The pandemic became Donald Trump's stage for "resilience performance", the manifestation of a healthy, powerful, and masculine identity of a political leader against the backdrop of a weaker, inferior and vulnerable Other (Bonacchi & Warnke, 2021). Since resilience in an individual can be interpreted as resilience in a group or a nation, in particular, then disease narratives became a convenient strategy for the self-representation of Trump's masculine resilience style and the assertion of his identity as the nation's leader (Bonacchi & Warnke, 2021, 58). Thus, Trump's disease discourse, marked by manifestations of masculine resilience, can be argued to represent a new form of "soft authoritarianism" and a threat to liberal democracy (Bonacchi & Warnke, 2021, 63).

The described local contexts, in which the measures to contain the epidemic were institutionally imposed, reveal a common dimension linked to the exercise of power and its validation at the level of discursive mechanisms. The anti-

COVID-19 measures, from restrictions on individual freedom to impositions and compulsory vaccination, required validation mechanisms at the discursive level. This task was entrusted to medical authorities, experts and politicians, giving rise to what has been called an "infodemic" (Cinelli et al., 2020). Especially in the first phase of the covidose emergency, "discursive authorities" in the sense of "ideology brokers" (Blommaert, 1999) emerged from the mainstream, i. e. from the centrality of the discourse, while the voices of protest were initially treated as a "periphery" (further on this aspect Warnke, Bonacchi & Seiler Bryll, 2023, 129). Soon, however, an increasing involvement of very heterogeneous protest groups was to be observed. This created a deep tension between centrality (power structures, traditional ideologies and the influence of the media) and marginality (those who are outside or on the margins of established structures). The reversal of positions occurs when marginalised groups begin to gain power through acts of protest, shifting and even reversing the mechanisms of power dynamics. This process is to be considered a part of a general movement oriented to questioning, criticising and at the end disrupting discursive orders (Meier-Vieracker et al., 2025). In the COVID-19 discourses, it is at this point that a subversion of epistemic (b)orders occurs, which means that alternative knowledge systems (with new frames, new borders, new mechanisms of inclusion and exclusion of paradigms etc.) begin to gain prominence and challenge the dominant forms of knowledge. This shift in knowledge structures is fundamental to the way in which power relations are renegotiated.

From the current perspective, we can observe some shifts when considering the interplay between various (institutional) actors in the field of vaccination and critical groups. While the general social body and its safety (solidified by medical and political institutions and their discursive manifestations) was the dominant point of reference both in the public debate and in vaccination rates, especially in the first phases of the COVID-19 pandemic, we can observe that after the initial activism phase, the opponents to vaccination trying to position themselves as an increasingly strong group and establish themselves as the group on which the safety of the social body can be made dependent, a state of affairs which has an influence on vaccination rates, which incidentally currently go much further than vaccinations against COVID-19. This example clearly shows the role of discursively mediated power and its influence on all non-discursive elements of our reality (here in the form of vaccination rates).

In retrospect, the COVID-19 pandemic can be considered from at least four perspectives: medical (institutionally led by the WHO), psychological, social and discursive. If we go one step further, it is possible to differentiate certain stages that capture the non-discursive (not least in the sense of power effects and in the sense of reality setup) and discursive dynamics of the COVID-19 pandemic.

From a medical point of view, eight phases were identified for the years 2020–2022 in many national contexts: Phase 0 (occurrence of sporadic cases), Phase 1 (first COVID-19 wave), Phase 2 (summer plateau 2020), Phase 3 (second COVID-19 wave), Phase 4 (summer plateau 2020), Phase 5 (fourth COVID-19 wave, VOC Delta), Phase 6 (fifth COVID-19 wave, Omicron BA. 1/ BA.2), and Phase 7 (sixth COVID-19 wave, VOC Omicron BA.5)[1]. Looking further ahead (2020–2029) and in relation to World Health Organisation documents intended as a strategy[2], the following three time frames can be distinguished:

- COVID-19 RESPONSE: Regional plans to reduce and control the incidence of SARS-CoV-2 infections and to prevent, diagnose and treat COVID-19 to reduce mortality, morbidity and long-term sequelae. In this phase, mass vaccination measures have been taken in the various countries affected by the pandemic. In these months, vaccination measures were taken in all countries;
- COVID-19 TRANSITION: Global and Regional plans to exit the COVID-19 emergency, to build on the response momentum, invest and institutionalise gains, kick-start stronger and more resilient health systems;
- PREPAREDNESS 2.0: a Regional Strategy and Action plan to bolster health emergency preparedness, response and resilience in the WHO European Region, according to what was already declared in the European Programme of Work (EPW) for 2020–2025.

Beyond this medical dimension, the pandemic had very incisive psychological effects at the level of individual and social behaviour. After an initial phase of restrained activism, in which people were united in facing the emergency of the pandemic, a phase of polarisation emerged, in which criticism and doubts became radicalised in the form of reactions to coercive measures to combat the pandemic, such as masks, compulsory vaccination, distancing, and restrictions on social life. In 2020, the following phases were identified[3], which relate to the way people faced the pandemic in their everyday life and in social interactions:

---

1 See for example Finne, Nowak & Razum, 2025.

2 "COVID-19 strategic preparedness and response plan : operational planning guidelines to support country preparedness and response: draft as of 12 February 2020" (https://digitallibrary.un.org/record/3859863?v=pdf (19 December 2024); "COVID-19 Strategic Preparedness and Response Plan 2022: Global Monitoring and Evaluation Framework"(https://www.who.int/publications/m/item/covid-19-strategic-preparedness-and-response-plan-2022-global-monitoring-and-evaluation-framework (19 December 2024); "Strategy and action plan on health emergency preparedness, response and resilience in the WHO European Region". (https://www.who.int/europe/teams/who-health-emergencies-programme-(whe)/preparedness-2.0 (19 December 2024).

3 https://www.land.nrw/sites/default/files/asset/document/rheingold_institut_-_die_phasen_der_corona-krise_aus_psychologischer_sicht.pdf (19 December 2024).

- Phase 1: Collective braking activism (see also Gerstenblatt, 2021). This phase is characterised by demonstrations of personal agency and solidarity with politicians. Politicians are seen as approachable crisis managers;
- Phase 2: Polarization phase. Doubts and polarised fronts emerge regarding attitudes to the COVID-19 pandemic, causing a division in perceptions of the reality of life in society. Everyday life becomes stressful as it slows down (see also van Bavel et al., 2024);
- Outlook for Phase 3: The outlining of strategies to construct differentiated paths to a "responsible normality" or a "new normality" (see also Manuti et al., 2022, Weidacher, 2025) is a challenge for all societies considered and a task above all for the political sphere.

Two important considerations arise at this point. On the one hand, many psychological aspects associated with COVID-19, such as shock, trauma or, more broadly, restriction of freedom (see Mustafa, 2021; Haas, 2021), have not been taken into account. On the other hand, and looking at the psychological phases from a contemporary perspective, we can see that phase 3, i. e. the construction of pathways to normality, should be considered in a more comprehensive way than just a return to the situation before the pandemic, in this sense a "neutralisation" of the pandemic is possible until the number of infections decreases. The aforementioned strong polarisation, which is central to the theme of this volume, has left little space for the negotiation of a socially and politically grounded normality. In the context of the COVID-19 pandemic, normality was a discursive figure between the expectation of a return to the pre-pandemic reality and the debate about the "new normality", which focused more on the consequences of the pandemic.

The observations outlined here open up a more socially oriented perspective. Among the most important aspects in this regard are social factors, which have exacerbated social inequality (globally and locally), which itself has paved the way for various polarisations. If we try to identify these, we can start with the observation that the debate on vaccination was initiated by a social and political expectation regarding a vaccine, which can also be seen in the categories of pressure and constriction. This was followed by hierarchisation within the social system, with prioritisation within COVID-19 vaccination recommendations being determined in many national contexts, i. e. certain population groups were given priority for voluntary vaccination. In the meantime, the first doubts about the vaccines arose, doubts which were linked in particular to their relatively rapid introduction and the lack of solid research regarding any negative consequences and side effects.

The protest against the COVID-19 vaccine (antivax, free vax or novax-movement) is to be considered as a very complex process in which three levels can be recognised. The first level concerns groups of vaccine opponents who were against all forms of vaccination, regardless of the COVID-19 pandemic. This very diverse group includes, for example, liberalists, people with religious motivations or ecologists (Crupi et al., 2022). The second group was made up of people who were not only AGAINST vaccination, but also against significant restrictions on unvaccinated people. They argued that unvaccinated people should not be discriminated against in social life. Beyond these two levels, we can identify a political level in which the fight against vaccination has become a political tool to gain power. It concerns all the political-strategic processes that sought to instrumentalise the growing power of the anti-vaccination movement for their own political interests and bore the hallmarks of a populist and alarmist discourse. (in a "weaponization of information", see Fominaya, 2022). The resulting extreme polarisation and the associated strengthening of anti-vaccination sentiments in the social arena also had medical consequences in the form of the transfer of this attitude to other types of vaccination.

From all these medical, psychological and social configurations in individual countries some key aspects emerge (in the case of the present volume, these are the discursive constructions in the area surrounding COVID-19), which opened the way for the articulation of different varieties of anti-vaccine discourse.

Let us now consider the characteristics that emerged in the discourse figurations analysed in this volume. The first striking feature is that anti-vaccine discourse is a global discourse characterised by locally determined polyvocality and extreme dynamicity (Duszak, House & Kumięga, 2010). Global and local are, in our volume, not spatial structures, but above all a dialectical realisation among discursive constructions of psychological, political and social reality that reveal certain epistemic orders. On the one hand, the contributors have tried to show the local logics of these discourses, concerning German (see Kumięga in this volume), American (see Godlewska in this volume) and Italian (see Bonacchi; Gobo; Campo & Serafini; Lello & Bertuzzi in this volume) perspectives, and, on the other hand, the universal and cohesive social and linguistic mechanisms. Of particular relevance to this publication are the microdiscursive aspects present in all the texts, aspects which address the specificity of the discursive constructions surrounding the COVID-19 pandemic discourse.

In an attempt to summarise the contributions contained in this volume, we are able to identify some characteristic elements of the analysed anti-vaccine discourses. At the level of agendas, we effectively have a structured polarisation in the argumentative struggle pro and contra the vaccine imposition that is based on oppositional systems of stance-taking, in which Othering all opponents is an essential element. On this basis, criteria of identity and group belonging are established. The arguments applied are sometimes scientific, sometimes dictated by common sense wisdom or power. In many cases, the arguments used are not rational, but based on "conspiracy theories" (see Czyżewski; Niehr in this volume), on widespread fears of "puppet masters" who hide behind pharmaceutical multinationals, capital groups, and lobby interests. In some cases, we can observe an attempted subversion of the cognitive (b)orders at the foundations of the various discourses: the (dis)information is not so much disseminated as reduplicated (see the contribution of Bonacchi in this volume), medical knowledge begins to falter not only due to the effect of fake news and pseudoscientific interventions but also due to internal dynamics in the circulation of expert knowledge (see the contributions of Gobo; Campo & Serafini in this volume). The downsizing of scientific culture and medical authority, the outbursts of anger and the acts of subversion, observed in many manifestations of the anti-vax movement, also express the rejection of classical rationality as a suspected neoliberal legacy. Specifically, anti-vaccine positions are mainly expressed in the refusal to vaccinate, in the sabotage of medical measures aimed at allowing vaccinations, in the refusal of the restrictions for not vaccinated people, and in the commitment to convince others and express one's dissent. From the point of view of the actors, we have the overlapping of authoritative institutional voices ("ideology brokers"), represented by doctors, politicians, experts, and the voices of people, often silenced, who claim for themselves the right to speak. It is a sort of "democratization 2.0" of the system of creating and guiding opinion, which now moves from the control of experts to the impact of influencers and average people who suddenly claim to have a "voice". Among them, "haters" stand out in particular (see Bonacchi's contribution in this volume). We also have many anonymous voices, which become depersonalised in ideology making. It is characteristic of the discourses that emerged during COVID-19, including the anti-vaccine discourse, that they led to the emergence of new discursive spaces and arenas. While public discourse uses all available means of information (mass media and digital spaces), protest movements often choose the streets to performatively demonstrate their criticism. The web remains the favorite channel of anti-vaccine movements where "digital squadrons" have been formed.

Let us end our considerations by returning to the motivation of the volume, which was to offer meta-discursive and meta-scientific reflections on the phenomenon analysed. That is, we asked ourselves, still in the midst of COVID-19, to what extent our discipline, namely linguistics and discourse analysis, is able to develop tools for acting on social reality. In this sense, our volume raises metalinguistic questions concerning the function of linguistic tools (see the contribution by Niehr; Kumięga in this volume), in particular discourse analysis instruments, to investigate complex social processes such as opinion-making and decision-taking processes, the formation of opposition and protest groups, the distrust of medical-scientific arguments and the propensity towards alternative logic systems.

More broadly, our volume also poses questions relating to the legitimacy of such analyses in the context of a discourse that, at the time of publication of this monograph, is not a discourse closed to its further linguistic, social and political dynamics (see the contribution by Warnke).

At this point, we would like to thank all the authors of the texts for accepting the invitation to reflect on various aspects of the anti-vaccine discourse, highlighting the interdisciplinary view of its linguistic constitution, immersed in its social and political dimensions. We would like to thank the authorities of the University of Gdańsk and the University of Warsaw for funding our project. Our thanks also go to the publisher of this volume, particularly for their editorial support.

Works cited

BBC, 2020. Coronavirus: Outcry after Trump suggests injecting disinfectant as treatment. *BBC* 24.04. bbc.com. (21 May 2024).

Blommaert, J. (1999). The debate is open. In J. Blommaert (ed.), *Language Ideological Debates* (pp. 1–38). Berlin, New York: De Gruyter Mouton.

Bonacchi, S. & Warnke, I.H. (2021). "We will go through this TOGETHER!" – Bemerkungen zu Vulnerabilität und zum kompulsiven Resilienzvarieté in politischen COVID-19-Krankheitsnarrativen. In D. Kaczmarek & J. Pędzisz (eds.), *Diskursive Spielräume des Gemeinsamen.* Lublin Studies in Modern Languages and Literature 45, 2, 2021, 53–64, DOI: 10.17951/lsmll.2021.45.1.53-64.

Bosen R.& Thurau, J. (2021). Chronology: How COVID has spread in Germany. https://www.dw.com/en/covid-how-germany-battles-the-pandemic-a-chronology/a-5802687 (12 December 2021).

Bradner E., Klein B. & Hickey C. (2021). Biden targets Trump's legacy with first-day executive Actions. *CNN* 20.01. https://edition.cnn.com/2021/01/20/politics/executive-actions-biden/index.html. (12 July 2025).

Bröckling, U. (2012). Dispositive der Vorbeugung: Gefahrenabwehr, Resilienz, Precaution. In C. Daase, P. Offermann & V. Rauer (eds.), *Sicherheitskultur. Soziale und politische Praktiken der Gefahrenabwehr* (pp. 93–108). Frankfurt/Main: Campus.

Chow, D. & Saliba, E. (2020). Italy has a world-class health system. The coronavirus has pushed it to the breaking point. *NBC News* 18.03. https://www.nbcnews.com/health/health-news/italy-has-world-class-health-system-coronavirus-has-pushed-it-n1162786 (03 August 2024).

Cinelli, M., Quattrociocchi, W., Galeazzi, A., Valensise, C.M., Brugnoli, E., Schmidt, A.L., Zola, P., Zollo, F. & Scala, A. (2020). The COVID-19 social media infodemic. *Scientific Reports* 10, 16598. https://www.nature.com/articles/s41598-020-73510-5 (28 February 2023).

Colgrove, J. K. (2006). *The State of Immunity. The Politics of Vaccination in Twentieth-Century.* America. Berkeley: University of California Press.

Coronaviridae Study Group of the International Committee on Taxonomy of Viruses. (2020). The species: Severe acute respiratory syndrome-related coronavirus: classifying 2019-nCoV and naming it SARS-CoV-2. *Nature Microbiology* 5, 536–544. https://doi.org/10.1038/s41564-020-0695-z (10 January 2024).

Crupi, G., Mejova, Y., Tizzani, M., Paolotti, D. & Panisson, A. (2022). Echoes through Time: Evolution of the Italian COVID-19 Vaccination Debate. *Proceedings of the International AAAI Conference on Web and Social Media*, 16, 1, 102–113. https://doi.org/10.1609/icwsm.v16i1.19276.

della Porta, D. & Lavizzari, A. (2022). Waves in cycle: The protests against anti-contagion measures and vaccination in COVID-19 times in Italy. *Partecipazione e Conflitto* 15, 3, 720–740.

Duszak, A., House, J. & Kumięga, Ł. (eds.) (2010). *Globalization, Discourse, Media: In a Critical Perspective.* Warszawa: Wydawnictwa Uniwersytetu Warszawskiego.

Finne, E, Nowak, A.C. & Razum, O. (2025). Regional COVID-19 measures and effects on subjective well-being in Germany: observing trends over time with data from a large population survey. *Front Public Health*, 27, 02,13, 1523691. doi: 10.3389/fpubh.2025.1523691. PMID: 40084213; PMCID: PMC11905229.

Fominaya, C.F. (2022). Mobilizing During the COVID-19 Pandemic: From Democratic Innovation to the Political Weaponization of Disinformation. *American Behavioral Scientist* 68, 6, 829–852.

Foucault, M. (2004). *Sicherheit, Territorium, Bevölkerung. Geschichte der Gouvernementalität I.* Frankfurt/Main: Verlag.

Gerstenblatt, P. (2021). What COVID-19 has brought us to: Art, activism, and changes in social work education. *Qual Soc Work*, 20.03. (1–2): 595–603. doi: 10.1177/1473325020973440. PMID: 34305460; PMCID: PMC8287082.

Haas, J.G. (2021). *COVID-19 and Psychology: People and Society in Times of Pandemic.* Germany: Springer Fachmedien Wiesbaden.

Inverardi, M. & Nienaber, M. (2020). Germany with over 1,100 cases, reports first two coronavirus deaths. *Reuters* 09.03. https://www.reuters.com/article/us-health-coronavirus-germany-death/germany-reports-first-death-cases-due-to-coronavirus-idUSKBN20W295/ (03 August 2024).

Jacobsen, G.D. & Jacobsen, K.H. (2020) Statewide COVID-19 Stay-at-Home Orders and Population Mobility in the United States. *World Medical & Health Policy*, 12, 12, 4, 347–356. https://www.ncbi.nlm.nih.gov/pmc/articles/PMC7405141/#wmh3350-bib-0023 (02 July 2024).

John Hopkins University Coronavirus Resource Center. Mortality Analyses. https://coronavirus.jhu.edu/data/mortality (02 July 2024).

Manuti, A., Van der Heijden, B., Kruyen, P., De Vos, A., Zaharie, M. & Lo Presti, A. (2022). Editorial: How Normal Is the New Normal? Individual and Organizational Implications of the COVID-19 Pandemic. *Front Psychol* 21, 06; 13:931236, doi: 10.3389/fpsyg.2022.931236. PMID: 35800919; PMCID: PMC9253824.

Meier-Vieracker, S. Acke, H., Bonacchi, S., Dang-Anh, M. & Warnke, I. H. (2025). Discourses in/of Disruption – An Introduction. In S. Meier-Vieracker, H. Acke, S. Bonacchi, M. Dang-Anh & I.H. Warnke (eds.), *Discourses in/of Disruption, Bd. 9 (Diskurs – interdisziplinär 12)*, IDS-Open 9, Manheim: IDS-Verlag, DOI: https://doi.org/10.21248/idsopen.9.2025.39.

Merkaj, E.& Santolini, R. (2022). Italian national policies in response to the COVID-19 pandemic: The case of the Friuli-Venezia-Giulia and Umbria Regions. *Health Policy*, Ap., 126, 4, 287–293. doi: 10.1016/j.healthpol.2022.02.004 (13 August 2024). https://www.ncbi.nlm.nih.gov/pmc/articles/PMC8874741/.

Mustafa, Ahmed A. (2021). *Mental Health Effects of COVID-19.* Netherlands: Academic Press.

Paterlini, M. (2020). On the Front Lines of Coronavirus: The Italian Response to COVID-19. BMJ 368: m1065. [PubMed] [Google Scholar]

Plümper, T., Neumayer, E. & Pfaff, K.G. (2021). The strategy of protest against COVID-19 containment policies in Germany. *Social Science Quarterly* 102, 5: 2236–2250.

Pustake, M., Tambolkar, I., Giri, P. & Gandhi, C. (2022). SARS, MERS and COVID-19: An Overview and comparison of clinical, laboratory and radiological features. *J Family Med Prim Care*, 31, 1, 1, 10–17. Retrieved 03 March 2024, from DOI: 10.4103/jfmpc.jfmpc_839_21.

Sheikh, K. (2020). No More Than 10 People in One Place, Trump Said. But Why?. *The New York Times*, 16, 3. ISSN 0362-4331. Archived from the original on August 28, 2020. https://nytimes.com (15 April 2023).

Thießen, M. (2017). *Immunisierte Gesellschaft. Impfen in Deutschland im 19. und 20. Jahrhundert.* Göttingen: Vandenhoeck & Ruprecht.

Tolksdorf, K., Loenenbach, A. & Buda, S. (2022). Dritte Aktualisierung der "Retrospektiven Phaseneinteilung der COVID-19-Pandemie in Deutschland". *Epid Bull*, 38, 3–6. doi:10.25646/10598.

Van Bavel, J.J., Pretus, C., Rathje, S., Pärnamets, P., Vlasceanu, M. & Knowles, E.D. (2024). The Costs of Polarizing a Pandemic: Antecedents, Consequences, and Lessons. *Perspectives on psychological science: a journal of the Association for Psychological Science*, 19, 4, 624–639. https://doi.org/10.1177/17456916231190395 (19 December 2024).

Wang, C., Horby, P.W., Hayden, F.G. & Gao, F.G. (2020). Novel coronavirus outbreak of global health concern. *The Lancet*, 395, 10223, 470–473. https://doi.org/10.1016/S0140-6736(20)30185-9 (15 February 2021).

Warnke, I., Bonacchi, S. & Seiler Brylla, Ch. (2023). Mimicry of Marginality – On Masking Hegemonic Positions Through Discourse. In *Mimicry of Marginality.* Special issue: *Zeitschrift für Diskursforschung.* Weinheim: Beltz Verlag, Juventa 2, 2023, 129–142.

Weidacher, G. (2025). Alte Normalität, neue Normalität. Die rhetorisch argumentative Verwendung des Begriffs *Normalität* während der Corona-Krise. In R. Opiłowski, H.E.H. Lenk, B. Mikołajczyk & N. Bentel (eds.), *Argumentation, Persuasion und Manipulation in Medientexten und -diskursen* (pp. 351–364). Göttingen: Vandenhoeck & Ruprecht.

Worldometers. (2024). "The official statistics about the death toll in the world". https://www.worldometers.info/coronavirus/#countries (14 February 2025).

Metadiscursive Considerations

Ingo H. Warnke

Vaccinated with Essayistic Words Against Flag-Waving Discourses – Traces of a Refusal

Abstract

The paper seeks an essayistic answer to the question of whether there are possibilities for a different scholarly discourse beyond polarising discourses that nevertheless makes contemporary political spaces analytically understandable. A hallmark of this pursuit is a refusal of the given topic. This is also evident in the style, which deliberately leaves behind conventional methods of scholarly presentation. The result is the study of questions about the COVID-19 pandemic and the so-called anti-vaxxers beyond one's own discursive entanglement in the topic. Or, in other words: this is precisely about taking into account the impossibility of writing about the COVID-19 pandemic without being positioned oneself. The paper is organised as a walk through the city and as a study in listening to music. The aim of the text is to dissipate flag-waving discourses through a radically different language.

Keywords: flag-waving discourses, walk through the city, listening to music, discourse analysis.

This essay is a non-text, or tries to be. It is characterised by an attitude of refusal. When scholarly texts are rejected for publication, they are not usually recognised by reviewers as scholarly achievements. This is different here. The present text does not itself claim to say anything about the given topic. This is done deliberately and intentionally.

I caution readers because this refusal makes for a complicated text. Confusion rather than clarity is sought here. It is a text that hesitantly approaches something, but then circles around and passes by, finally finding itself completely out in the open. A text that does not want to arrive anywhere. A text about music that one hears in passing. A text that holds back strict academic sense and, at the same time, does not address those who doubt strict scholarship. An essay that visits an exhibition and speaks again and again of the traces of a refusal or rejection and becomes entangled in paradoxes.

Ingo H. Warnke, University of Bremen, ORCID: 0009-0008-6948-8426.

This text is a kind of self-vaccination against flag-waving[1] discourses. Outraged publics waving flags, old and new flags, are deeply suspicious to me and they meet my utter rejection. I know that in doing so, I am not doing outrage itself any favours, and I may be criticising it too quickly. I know that my words run the risk of discriminating against outrage. I know that Stéphane Hessel (2011) attributes to outrage the power to produce resistance. And I know that he refers to the Résistance, to National Socialism, and to decolonisation. And I know that I don't want to question resistance in principle, ever. But these are not flag-waving discourses in my understanding. Contemporary historical revisionism, hostility to science, anti-democratic habitus, hate speech, all the unsavoury figurations of zealous masses: this is flag-waving.

There will be no research question in this text and no reliable findings. And yet many questions will be asked, answers will at least be sought. Here and there, the text will confront questions about the so-called *anti-vaxxers*, opponents of vaccination. But I will explicitly not seek to answer them. There are two simple reasons for this: (i) I do not want to participate in a re-enactment of the debates by and around anti-vaxxers as they were conducted in the heyday of the COVID-19 pandemic because I do not want to valorise the argumentative topoi of anti-science discourses by paying attention to them in a discourse-linguistic publication, and (ii) I consider the topic obsolete by now and, in light of other pressing issues, I aim to give no stage to the theater of fools that probably exists in every epoch.

... This text could begin in this or any similar way and end right here.

But perhaps it is worthwhile following at least one trace. Therefore, I will take the set task seriously.

The theme of this contribution[2] gestures toward a discursive tension, we could also say toward the contradiction of positions between supporters and opponents of compulsory vaccination in the context of the COVID-19 pandemic. What I am called to do is to ask about the *who*, *what*, and *how* of the opponents of vaccination. I am asked to address *who* the vaccination opponents are as a group of self-identification, *what* they make the object of their knowledge worlds, and *how* they do this communicatively.

But why is there any interest at all in the social figure of the anti-vaxxer? What does this interest say about those who ask about it, about the relationship between this figure and those they ask about it?

1 See https://www.rbb24.de/politik/thema/2020/coronavirus/beitraege_neu/2020/10/fahnen-anti-corona-bewegung-demonstrationen.html (16 April 2023).

2 I refer here to the cfp of the online workshop *The Green Pass Conflict: Wer, was, wo und wie? Die "No Vax(ers)" in Deutschland, Italien und Polen*, organized by the University of Warsaw and the Silesian University of Technology, which took place on 17–18 February 2022.

Although these questions are not uninteresting in general, I will neither address them explicitly, nor focus on the discourse-linguistic question of *how*. I certainly recognise the anti-vaxxer – generically speaking – as a significant figure in COVID-19 discourse. Of course, one can also ask how this figure acts linguistically, how it positions itself in relation to the pandemic through a specifically constructed concept of truth, and not least, how it is positioned in metafigurative discourses as an opponent of vaccination.[3]

We can deal with all of this, but why should we do so? What deontic logic is at work here?

Hasn't the figure of the anti-vaxxer long since become passé, perhaps even forgotten, at the latest when someone takes this text into their hands, just like the flâneur takes a book into their hands in a small library on the fringes of metropolitan bustle? Wasn't the figure of the anti-vaxxer created above all for fleeting resonances of media attention in the first place?

Why should I bother with this any further? Today, when vaccination certificates only have their hidden digital presence in apps of old smartphones and are updated no longer, and when we might have a sheet of old paper lying around here or there, with a QR code that no longer refers to anything? Because we hope to learn something, that would be the obvious answer. Because an interest in the figure of the anti-vaxxer makes it an object of scholarly observation, another answer. And because thereby, observing scholarly subjects distance themselves from their objects. This is probably the point: the core of the set task. A gesture of distancing is requested.

To work discourse-linguistically on the figure of the anti-vaxxer seems to me first and foremost a project of distancing. What is to be said in this project, what deontic logics of the sayable are pursued by it, what supposed obligatoriness is associated with it? I think this is about a scholarly defense reflex against the science denialism of certain discursive configurations in the COVID-19 pandemic. I could understand such a reflex. But why *should* I follow it? Is the analysis of non-shared attitudes – I myself have been vaccinated and boosted and recovered – a compulsory task of discourse analysts because there are issues on which we should take a stance, because there are deontic rules structuring the sayable? This is arguably not at all about the question of what I can say or what others supposedly cannot say, this is not at all about possibilities but about reflexes, effects, and about acknowledging a must that appears in discourse.

This would mean, however, that the motivation to deal with the topic posed here is part of the same discursive formation as that which should be observed.

3 See *Neuer Wortschatz rund um die Coronapandemie:* https://www.owid.de/docs/neo/listen/corona.jsp (04 April 2023).

But where does this leave questions of scholarly distance? In other words, I don't want to say anything at all about the deontic questions raised here. I distance myself from the super-presentness of a comprehensible reflex and thus to the super-reactivity of the humanities in general, and I distance myself from a scholarly habitus that radically realises the present.

Probably, my philological training simply stands in the way. I prefer to branch out into the details of the Grimm's woods, to remain fragmentary, rather than rising to a diagnosis of the present with the great levers of universal discourse. Or is this rather a matter of refusing to follow the reflex against flag-waving? Do I aim to avoid contact with a world that is remote from me?

In any case, my refusal also results from a critique of a reflex that converts publics of the present into scholarly capital. What bothers me about this is the paradigm of reactive production. The impulse to immediately write a paper about those who stand in the street with their cardboard signs and question liberal democracy. I refuse to accept an all-pervasive logic of production in the scholarly attentions of the present; more generally, I am sceptical of "the obsession with production alone" (Latour & Schultz, 2022, no page).

It is obvious, however, that I am entangled in a pragmatic contradiction through my own production of this text. But indeed, I doubt the scholarly value of comprehensible reflexes, in which what has just been seen is already converted into products, into scholarly capital. The figure of the anti-vaxxer seems – putting this cynically – almost welcome, because it is quickly convertible into procedures of scholarly production. In the end, we can congratulate ourselves on papers, books, talks, and scripts: the figure of the anti-vaxxer has become a commodity. Following this market logic, the aforementioned deontic logics are nothing else but the demonstration of the possibility of increasing scholarly capital by countering current science denialism.

This reminds me of Theodor W. Adorno's remarks on the marketing of the essay as a superficial product for customers, a scholarly gesture of autonomy thus liberating itself into unfreedom: "Torn itself [sic!] becomes unfree and sets itself to work in the service of the socially performed needs of its customers" (Adorno, 1958/1984, 154).

I see scholarly work critically where it fulfils customer needs and is committed to a logic of production – even if this results from ethically noble reflexes. I try to evade an obligation to produce corresponding products. I step aside and prefer to listen to music in the precious remainder of life time. For example, Caroline Shaw (*1982), her *Three Essays* for string quartet. An occasion of this music is the year 2016, for the composer a year "deeply troubled by the national unrest leading to and resulting from that year's presidential election."[4] This music, these three

4 See: https://www.hyperion-records.co.uk/dw.asp?dc=W22095_120650 (21 April 2023).

musical essays are obviously also a reaction to the present, but one that is far removed from scholarly logics of exploitation.

The fragmentary composition, in parts beautiful, in other parts disturbing, which takes a running start again and again and at the same time retreats again and again, breaking out here and there, "premiered […] at the BBC Proms in 2018."[5] *Three Essays* "address language's power to stir emotion and spread information and ideas through written, spoken and digital forms."[6] They are about information and confusion of discourse: "Much like in the COVID-19 epidemic, she [Caroline Shaw] saw language being used to spread information about current events but also, and increasingly, to spread confusion and misinformation."[7]

How to respond linguistically to the fact that language is used to confuse and misinform? Within the framework of scholarly market logics?

I hear the music as refusal, and I have arrived, like Caroline Shaw, at the essay. Adorno (1958/1984, 152) helps me to understand why: "The essay, however, does not permit its domain to be prescribed. Instead of achieving something scientifically, or creating something artistically, the effort of the essay reflects a childlike freedom that catches fire, without scruple, on what others have already done." This matches my textual refusal. Like anti-vaxxers obtain their figuration from contradicting, I also stage myself in lines of an against. However, I do so on the other side, this side of scholarship, not beyond it; one must not confuse the two.

This provides a first answer to the question of what texts – like this one – say about those who write them. They are obviously on the other side, this side, in scholarship. That is the place of my voice as well, and I share that place, I assume, with all those who have contributed to this book. Persons who belong to scholarship and who are concerned about the foolish fashion of a hostility toward science and scholarship.

But what cannot be overlooked is that this place is also a place of privilege. Neither has the pandemic significantly restricted me in my activities, nor have I experienced any hardships due to it, neither materially nor psychologically. I live in the privilege of the knowledge producers who are institutionally validated, which does not mean that I am privileged everywhere and in principle, of course. But my point of view in writing about non-vaccinated people is that of a privileged distance. I am a trained philologist and have learned to operate at this distance, in that sense, this is nothing unusual. But what does this distance do to the subject matter assigned here, the question of the discourses of the unvacci-

5 See: https://www.hyperion-records.co.uk/dw.asp?dc=W22095_120650 (21 April 2023).
6 See: https://www.hyperion-records.co.uk/dw.asp?dc=W22095_120650 (21 April 2023).
7 See: https://www.hyperion-records.co.uk/dw.asp?dc=W22095_120650 (31 March 2023).

nated? It others them and is thus part of an order of knowledge of split societies. But this inside and outside, this here and there, may be perceivable within the sharp boundaries of discourse, but that does not mean that these demarcations are unambiguous in everyday life. The picture is much more diffuse there. As soon as I get to know a vaccination sceptic, for example, and deal with their arguments, the boundaries become more permeable. If this person is a scientist themselves, even more so. Could it be, then, that the distance of one's position is primarily a sought-after imagination that has the purpose of mapping discourses in unambiguous ways?

Discourse analysis demands distance. Foucault's concept of the *archive* in its entanglement with *dispositif* and *discourse* is crucial here.

The Archeology of Knowledge states that the archive is "first the law of what can be said, the system that governs the appearance of statements as unique events" (Foucault, 1969/1972, 129). What could interest us more in the discourse of the unvaccinated than the question of the law of the appearance of certain statements? What is it that makes people say this or that at a time and thus adopt this or that attitude? Which dispositif makes the emergence of certain statements possible? As a working concept, dispositif can be understood with Constanze Spieß (2013, 18) as an "infrastructure or interaction framework for discourse". The *archive*, then, is the rule of sayables, the *dispositif* an infrastructure for linguistic and non-linguistic statements in an order of knowledge, and *discourse* the material and, in my understanding, linguistic manifestation of knowledge as encountered in individual statements but networked transtextually.

Which possibilities of the appearance of statements in an infrastructure of knowledge would we have to discuss? Here one should not overlook a methodological reminder by Foucault; I take it seriously. It says in *the Archeology of Knowledge:*

> The description of the archive deploys its possibilities (and the mastery of its possibilities) on the basis of the very discourses that have just ceased to be ours; its threshold of existence is established by the discontinuity that separates us from what we can no longer say, and from that which falls outside our discursive practice; it begins with the outside of our own language (*langage*); its locus is the gap between our own discursive practices. (Foucault, 1969/1972, 130–131)

So here, too, we are talking about a distance, a discontinuity. But it is precisely this distance that I do not have from the pandemic, despite all my privileges. Especially since these privileges were precisely those derived from the pandemic situation, such as the possibility of being able to work at home without further worries. Perhaps I even considered the pause of a lockdown as something to be welcomed; as the Nobel Prize in Literature laureate Olga Tokarczuk (2020) puts it.

What does that mean for this text here? I can either imagine a distance in discourse analysis and distance myself as a scholarly subject, or I reject the idea of working on non-vaccinated people. To me, the second stance seems more convincing. At least as a discourse linguist I reach my limits here. I am reminded of another historically grown imagination of distance. The glaring misconception that the postcolonial situation is a matter of Black people, the (formerly) colonised, the descendants of the enslaved, victimised subjects. But this distance does not exist either. The privileges of the whites, the former colonisers and their descendants, result from colonialism and thus whiteness is in the midst of the postcolonial constellation, not on the outside. This is arguably comparable with generations of victims and perpetrators of National Socialism.

So, is the reference to Foucault's concept of the archive too facile after all? Does the entanglement of a white position in the colonial history of violence, the lack of distance, in fact mean that there are no possibilities for whites to describe the colonial archive because the discourses that emerge from that archive persist? Does this cessation of discourse exist anywhere at all, this discursive line? What exactly is the gap Foucault is talking about? Is it not the case, rather, that all preceding discourses are woven into what I say? Is it not the case that the outside of our own discourses always exists only to a limited extent? It is, after all, the characteristic of any discourse that it can become ours again and again with a certain unpredictability, not least because texts can always be re-actualised.

But back to the non-vaccinated. Can I ever analyse the archive of their discourse production with their specific communicative infrastructures, that is, dispositifs, then? Starting from Foucault, I expect that a distance must open up between me and the object of investigation, a double movement: the subjectification of the researcher and the objectification of their subject.

But what if this distance actually does not exist because the discourses are ongoing and because I, as a researcher, find myself in the same situation of knowledge (if not in the same constellation of knowledge) as the researched? Then, discourse analysis would not be possible. Or the lack of distance implicitly (if not preconsciously) motivates an interest in writing about something that one cannot actually write about by constructing the distance of one's own position through one's writing and thereby inventing and positioning oneself as a researching subject.

I am stepping outside the door, putting on my headphones, and listen to the first essay by Caroline Shaw. Groping chords, the music is breaking off again and again, everything unfolds from a simple idea, impulses of movement. A cantilena in the cello, the music drives forward. But the simple things are getting more and more complicated, as in my lyrics, the music is getting caught up in itself. At some point, the music finds its way back to a grand harmony of individual, small fragments, like memories of a time when there could have been no distance. And the impulse of movement of the beginning returns. Stepping out of a messy situation, going ahead. In its ostinato monotony, the music is like a maelstrom, ending in great restlessness, agitation, in a disturbing glissando somewhere.

This first movement from the *Three Essays* is titled *Nimrod*. This also places us in the midst of the world of discourses. Caroline Shaw's music here is perhaps nothing more than a resonant metaphor for the impulses of movement in discourses and their unreliability. Nimrod's trace leads to the Tower of Babel (see Köller, 2012, 239–242), that archetype of human hubris and the confusion of languages: "In the Jewish and Christian literature of antiquity, N[imrod] is identified with the builder of the Tower of Babel and considered to be a sacrilegious person"[8]. But even given this mythical accusation, I might wonder if the discourses of hubris and of the fragmentation of an understanding of each other have ever ceased, if the archive of fragmentations is not as current as it has always been. Is Caroline Shaw's music actually a commentary on the present, I wonder, or on the ongoing disorder of discourse?

Keane (2020, 219) goes so far as to speak of an "infecting and degrading language" in describing new despotisms. It must indeed outrage us as scholars when we see the hatred of some anti-vaxxers, hear their hateful language, and their distance to reason. I listen to Shaw and am reminded by the name Nimrod of a distance which is anything but static or even reliable, which is surrounded by a great restlessness: flag-waving discourses. Perhaps these discourses are far away enough from me to dissect them ethically after all. However, these discourses have not stopped because they have never belonged to me in the first place, they have always been external to me.

Why do I have to listen to music, go out into town?

The answer is simple: because I have arrived at the essay. Because only in the genre of the essay can I encounter the task of writing about the non-vaccinated. And this was the requested task. Only the essay is radical enough: "radically unradical in refraining from any reduction to a principle, in accentuating the fragmentary, the partial rather then [sic!] the total" (Adorno, 1958/1984, 157).

And only in this fragmentary is it possible for me to capture something of what seems important enough to write about here. So I follow the course through the city, continue to listen to music, and circle the essay around the question of why one should work in a discourse-analytical framework about the non-vaccinated. One realisation has already emerged in the process: I am in the midst of discourses. I cannot look at the discursive grid of the pandemic dispositif from the outside, because I myself occupy a crossing point in it.

8 See: https://referenceworks.brillonline.com/entries/brill-s-new-pauly/nimrod-e823520 (08 April 2023).

It is true that the pandemic has lost attention by now. I no longer move in it in real time. But the subject matter itself continues to be intertwined with the discursive order of the pandemic. This is already evident from the fact that (critical) writing about the unvaccinated or vaccination critics and anti-vaxxers is associated with the implicature of one's own vaccination status. I can only see non-vaccinated people as a problem when I am vaccinated myself. But pondering over the unvaccinated as a vaccinated person is anything but reflecting the pandemic from a distance. It is, on the contrary, a perpetuation of a division within an order that was drawn as a discursive rift of the pandemic.

Overall, I am less interested in the concrete situation than in the discourse-theoretical and also the heuristic status of the problem. So with respect to my own positioning, I remain on the privileged side. Since I understand language as a finite, because power-bound and thus limited, realisation and processing of potentially infinite possibilities of utterances, the issue is therefore one of limitations. But if the archive as a rule of the sayable is what limits possible utterances, then I have to note that it does the same with my own discursive practices. As long as I find myself in the archive, I cannot look at it from the outside, nor can I look from outside at the discourses that it produces.

If an archival interest in language in fact presupposes distance, one can of course ask how much. Does this have to be an absolute distance, or is a relative distance already sufficient for analysis? Might a very small estrangement even be enough? For example, if I were to feed language data into a corpus, perhaps this abstraction would already be enough to distance it from discourse. Or is this a matter of years? How many years of time apart would be enough? One generation, one human life? (see Kämper, 2018, 54) And does it not already constitute a distance that I, as a vaccinated person, speak about so-called anti-vaxxers? It would then be necessary for evidentiary reasons, however, to disclose one's immunisation records. Do I really want this? And do the vaccinated and anti-vaxxers then really move in different archives; no: I had already come to realise that. More questions than answers.

And this brings me back to the increasingly clear realisation that the whole enterprise is questionable. Because: discourses do not really come to an end. So, this could merely be about working on a discursive polarisation that already exists. If I wanted to speak out of this polarisation at all (which is not the case), however, another trap would arise from the quote by Foucault. Let us take a second close look: "The description of the archive deploys its possibilities (and the mastery of its possibilities) on the basis of the very discourses that have just ceased to be ours [...]" (Foucault, 1969/1972, 130). But if I were to focus on the archive of the pandemic with critical intent and continued polarisation, then precisely the opposite would be true; then the discourses that should be at stake would never have been mine. In fact, only questionable conclusions can be drawn from this quotation. Either the discourses continue to belong to me, in which case I would not be able to describe the rules of their production at all, or the discourses under investigation did not belong to me in the first place, in which case, however, it would not be possible for me to understand the rules of their production either. Foucault's thought arguably is: should you want to describe and understand the archive, the discourses should have belonged to you in the past. How often is this the case? Much rather, it is the case that we are interested in rules of the sayable that we imagine as already external to us and that we (want to) criticise, or that we continue to be part of the discursive order of the subject matters that interest us.

In addition, the COVID-19 biopolitical archive is more comprehensive than the subject position of so-called anti-vaxxers: vaccination advocates, anti-vaxxers, vaccines and their development, vaccination centres, intensive care units, so-called corona walks, apps, contact restrictions, hygiene measures, restaurants, vaccination passports, corona measures, access rules, masks, trucker protests, and much more; all this has produced, in a dispositif mesh of bodies, materialities, and utterances, a certain formation of statements that one might then be tempted to call the discursive order of the anti-vaxxers.

Two sentences by Adorno come to mind here, with which he apodictically dissects the essay: "The relevance of the essay is that of anachronism" (Adorno, 1958/1984, 170). We have already noticed the outdated nature of the whole endeavour about the unvaccinated: to write, after the pandemic, about a subject matter that was considered with interest during the pandemic, taking a distance that is questionable, because it would be a distance today that one already had at that time, or precisely a persistent absence of any distance. All this calls for a certain aimlessness in writing. So I am poking around in some discursive pulp because even this is still surrounded by the promise of a scholarly aura. But in truth, I don't see why I should pursue a serious project here to begin with: "The essay, however, has to do with that which is blind in its objects" (Adorno, 1958/1984, 170).

So I keep listening to music, the second movement of Caroline Shaw's *Three Essays*. The title of the movement is *Echo*. An unsettling, rearing noise that rises in chords. A small, sad Bartók-like melody breaks out. All in all, however: single monotony. A short flicker also that does not trigger any movement. The chords finally blur into one another, no way out, the deceptive harmony of the final chord like the result of some kind of weird artificial intelligence. What comes to my mind, guided by the title, is the concept of the echo chamber[9]: "Social media may limit the exposure to diverse perspectives and favor the formation of groups of like-minded users framing and reinforcing a shared narrative, that is, echo

9 See https://www.hyperion-records.co.uk/dw.asp?dc=W22095_120650 (31 March 2023).

chambers" (Cinelli et al., 2021, 1). I imagine the anti-vaxxers in such echo chambers. There is something disturbing to which Caroline Shaw's music points here, an audible picture of missing perspectives. When parts of social media sound like this music, they make one feel frosty.

While I am walking through the city and thinking about the music, I come to stand in front of a gallery, see bookshelves, some books in them, as if it were the studio of a diligent student working on their doctoral thesis. An archive of searching investigation. I'm stepping in.

Now I am sitting here, in a small box surrounded by shelves. In the *C& Center of Unfinished Business* at the ifa Gallery Berlin.[10] It is a "reading room offering visitors an extraordinary, sometimes disconcerting selection of books that are linked to the topic of colonialism in various ways".[11] I am taking a look around. Maybe this would be a good place to write this text. A box in the middle of the city. A metaphorical place for the distance I need to occupy from those I am supposed to be dealing with: the anti-vaxxers. But before I start writing, I prefer to look around. I pick up a book from the shelf, open it: I read *Essay* as a title on the page. That captivates me right away. The text is written by Carsten Junker (2011), which captivates me even more. I cannot escape the essay. Just as I cannot escape the discourses that surround me, because I am caught up in the postcolonial situation that the words, books, and writings here tell us about, that reveal it, that make it impossible to overlook, if one looks behind the window pane and enters the archive of a persistent knowledge.

I wonder once again what Foucault means when he speaks *of the very discourses that have just ceased to be ours.* There is no trace of stopping here, and I also think again of the anti-vaxers and wonder now whether it is not they who want to build a distance to me. And whether it is not this will that persists, a discursive action of distancing that wants to declare me an elite to be fought. The key here is not to be evasive. I should perhaps begin to engage in enduring: enduring my entanglement in discourses and being addressed by acts of discourse.

In the last few years I have repeatedly been dealing with texts from the German colonial period. When I read these, I am often struck by utterances that are so completely foreign to me. I do not share their presuppositions, nor the manner of their expression. And it is here that I encounter the colonial archive, in a Foucauldian sense. The colonial discourse fragments are graspable for me as expressions of a law of historical possibilities and necessities of utterance, because they are not my discourse. The colonial archive is that which is separated from

10 See: https://www.ifa.de/ausstellung/contemporary-and-center-of-unfinished-business/ (31 March 2023).

11 See: https://contemporaryand.com/center-of-unfinished-business/ (31 March 2023).

my present; it contains that which I do not say (anymore), its place is the distance of discourses from the place of my language. And yet these discourses have not ceased at all. So perhaps I believe myself to be all too deceptively safe when I think that these discourses are not mine. Looking at it closely, I am moving into a contradiction here. Into a paradox: on the one hand, I think I understand what is meant when it is said that archival analysis, or in other words, the analysis of the modality of utterance, presupposes a distance, which I have, and on the other hand, I have to realise once again that I do not possess this very distance at all, because I am structurally involved in the persistence of the postcolonial world.

And it is precisely this paradox of distance, of acting in a distance that is proximity, that makes up the attempt to write about the anti-vaxxers. Whoever distances themselves from whom in the process: as a subject of research, I am always already part of the orders of knowledge of those who are supposedly so clearly different – all at the same time.

Can we understand the rules of sayability in discourses when we ourselves are within the boundaries of the very same rules? I think so, but it is important to pay particular attention here and ask ourselves where the distances are. The fact that I act on this side of scholarship and responsibility for others arguably opens up such a distance.

This does not mean, however, that I want to answer to the call for a deontics of sayability, an obligatoriness. I do not analyse the language of those who set themselves apart from my pandemic world, who position themselves so far away with their cardboard signs that outrage me. I am still repelled by the recollections of the protests back then. Of course, this would have given me just the distance that Foucault seems to have in mind.

So what is it that keeps me away? Why don't I, like others, work with the tools of discourse analysis to take on a task, to criticise flag-waving discourses with the tools of scholarship, and thus, perhaps, to stand in solidarity with those who seem to have been caught in the crosshairs of an angry crowd? I don't want to write about anti-vaxxers. But why on earth not?

The reason is that I am pursuing an auto-ethnographic project here, in which I have to deal with my own positions and ask questions:

- What are my privileges, do they get in the way or are they the necessary condition for my analysis?
- Where is my distance, where is the distance of others?
- Am I inside the discourse or indeed beside it or even beyond it?
- Has the discourse at issue already ceased or does it continue and shape my own scholarly practice?

I recognise more and more clearly that it is not the analysis that I am unwilling or unable to provide, but the speed of response that scholarly discourse here expects of me. But I am not a journalist and not a seismograph of my present. Others can do this much better. I am a philologically trained scholar of distance. And I am close to Foucault's words with my work. I take an engaged distance to the super-presentness of a comprehensible reflex and thus to the super-reactivity of scholarship in general. I am not part of those who academically strive for radically presenting the present.

So I go forward and move the doubts expressed. It is obvious that this results in a text that does little but defy the task at hand. Perhaps this is also an escape from a present that frightens me. Perhaps those who want to stand firm are more courageous. But perhaps my doubt is much more the paradoxical gesture of a massive contradiction against discourses that wave with flags and that want to teach us fear, us who stand on this side of some imagined, fragile certainty.

No: I do not analyse you. I pass by you, by your angry faces, by your zeal, by your self-painted signs! Your flags are not mine. Precisely because I cannot simply step out of the discourses, I drift out of the situation (see Storch & Warnke, 2020). So I go on.

I listen to the third movement of Caroline Shaw's *Three Essays*. It is titled *Ruby*. At first, the same confusion as with *Echo*. But then all of a sudden, an impulse of movement, a direction, a possibility seems to open up to find our way out of the sounds of shifted confusion. This is not an easy undertaking. It takes time. But then a figure is outlined from the fragments, a seven-step trajectory. Things remain complicated, but the tonal shape keeps making its way. With *Ruby*, are we in the clutches of a programming language or are we encountering the beauty of a gemstone?[12] It all ends in great turmoil, in trivial excitement, in a simple lamentation of a cold outside. With a final metallic chord.

I read a scathing review of this music, for whom what is heard here is "a complete compositional irrelevance and a total waste of time."[13] And I wonder where the coldness of these words comes from, which are even colder than the music itself. Perhaps these words are exactly what this music is about. I continue to drift out. Balked at the assignment to write something about the anti-vaxxers, but not from writing. I have picked up a trace: so much preferred my *irrelevance* and possible *total waste of time* to engaging with flag wavers on the streets of outrage with their black-white-red or other flags ready for violence, and thinking that this would be relevant and time well spent.

I turn away. I have cautioned against this: this text refuses to perform what is expected of it. But it is doing something quite active: it drifts out into the open,

12 See: https://www.hyperion-records.co.uk/dw.asp?dc=W22095_120650 (31 March 2023).

13 See: https://5against4.com/2018/07/19/proms-2018-caroline-shaw-second-essay-echo-third-essay-ruby-world-premieres/ (16 April 2023).

into flaglessness – the knowledge in which Foucault is interested is itself without origin and contingent (see Ebeling, 2020, 256).

In the end, one thing remains: I distance myself from distance, expose myself to uncomfortable discourses. Albeit via detours, following other thoughts than initially suspected. On walks through the city that take me to places where I only encounter more and more discourses. Listening to music – *Nimrod, Echo, Ruby* – that draws me into more discourses. Nothing has ceased. The only hold is the holdless essay itself, are my words in the essay. And so: I have vaccinated myself with these essayistic words while following the traces of a refusal.

Works cited

Adorno, T.W. (1958/1984). The Essay as Form. *New German Critique*, 32, 151–171.

Cinelli, M., G. De Francisci Morales, Galeazzi, A., Quattrociocchi, A. & Starnini, M. (2021). The Echo Chamber Effect on Social Media. *Proceedings of the National Academy of Sciences*, 118, 9. https://doi.org/10.1073/pnas.2023301118 (22 January 2022).

Ebeling, K. (2020). Archiv. In C. Kammler, R. Parr, & U. Schneider (eds.), *Foucault Handbuch. Leben – Werk – Wirkung* (256–57). Berlin: Metzler.

Foucault, M. (1969/1972). *The Archaeology of Knowledge*. New York: Pantheon. [Orig. *L'archéologie du savoir*. Paris: Gallimard.]

Hessel, S. (2011). *Time for Outrage!* London: Quartet Books.

Junker, C. (2011). Essay. In S. Arndt, & N. Ofuatey-Alazard (eds.), *Wie Rassismus aus Wörtern spricht: (K)Erben des Kolonialismus im Wissensarchiv der deutschen Sprache. Ein kritisches Nachschlagewerk* (pp. 272–84). Münster: Unrast.

Keane, J. (2020). *The New Despotism*. Cambridge/MA, London: Harvard UP.

Kämper, H. (2018). Diskurslinguistik und Zeitgeschichte. In I.H. Warnke (ed.), *Handbuch Diskurs* (pp. 53–74). Berlin, Boston: de Gruyter.

Köller, W. (2012). *Sinnbilder für Sprache. Metaphorische Alternativen zur begrifflichen Erschließung von Sprache*. Berlin, Boston: de Gruyter.

Latour, B. & Schultz. N. (2022). *On the Emergence of an Ecological Class – A Memo*. Cambridge, UK: Polity. [Orig. *Mémo sur la nouvelle classe écologique. Comment faire émerger une classe écologique consciente et fière d'elle-même*. Paris: Editions La Découverte.]

Shaw, C. (2020). Three Essays. Calidore String Quartet – Babel, Track 5–7. Signum Classics | SIGCD650.

Spieß, C. (2013). Texte, Diskurse und Dispositive. Zur theoretisch-methodischen Modellierung eines Analyserahmens am Beispiel der Kategorie Schlüsseltext. In K.S. Roth, & C. Spiegel (eds.), *Angewandte Diskurslinguistik: Felder, Probleme, Perspektiven* (17–42). Berlin: Akademie.

Storch, A. & Warnke. I.H. (2020). Sansibarzone. Eine Austreibung aus der neokolonialen Sprachlosigkeit. Bielefeld: transcript.

Tokarczuk, O. (2020). Jetzt kommen neue Zeiten! *Frankfurter Allgemeine Zeitung*, 31. 03; 77, 9.

Marek Czyżewski

Communicative Aspects of Conspiracy Theories

Abstract
The rationale for this paper is the conspicuous contrast between the immense persuasive force of conspiracy theories (including recent COVID-19 conspiracy theories) and an insufficient meta-reflection upon the state of their scholarly analyses. Against this backdrop, an attempt is undertaken to combine an analysis of conspiracy theories with a meta-analysis of scholarly theorizing on conspiracy theories. In view of the dominance of psychological research and theorizing on conspiracy theories and the high level of schematism in this field, a shift of scholarly interest is suggested toward an analysis of conspiratorial culture. Consequently, both conspiracy theories themselves and the theories of conspiracy theories are investigated in terms of their communicative features. More specifically, a brief outline of COVID-19 conspirational rhetoric is presented, resulting from the application of Fantasy Theme Analysis, one of the approaches in the domain of rhetorical criticism. In addition, some practical recommendations are formulated regarding advisable and inadvisable ways of talking about pandemic related issues. Apart from psychological and cultural-rhetorical perspectives, a third line of research is briefly introduced with reference to the interpretive current in social sciences.

Keywords: conspiracy theories, theories of conspiracy theories, COVID-19, conspirational culture, conspirational rhetoric, Fantasy Theme Analysis.

1. Introduction

Set before this text are two objectives. On the one hand, the latest wave of conspiracy theories – those associated with the COVID-19 pandemic alongside those associated with a broad range of (new and old, local and global) political clashes – calls for reflection upon the characteristics of and conditions for such theories in general. On the other hand, however, the significant upsurge in academic literature on conspiracy theories calls for a meta-reflection upon the current state of scholarly analyses on this topic. This article will therefore strive to tackle both

Marek Czyżewski, University of Łódź, ORCID: 0000-0001-9544-1420.

sides of this problem, but also attempt to bring to a nexus the issues the two present.

The first, concrete, and historically-situated problematics are connected with a certain paradox. At the threshold of the coronavirus pandemic, hopes were high that the need for a scientific diagnosis of the biological aspects of the contagion would create a chance for academia's importance to rise in public debate and, by the same token, for a new public enlightenment to take shape. It promptly turned out that such expectations were not only overly optimistic, but also simply naïve. Inasmuch as the pandemic did, in fact, arouse an immediate and immense mobilization, accelerate development of scientific research into the traits of this Coronaviridae virus, and expedite the derivation of the most feasibly effective vaccine, the outbreak of this pernicious disease did not in the least lead to a rationalization of the public sphere. Quite the contrary, COVID-19 opened a real window of opportunity for a boom in (it would seem) even the most absurd conspiracy theories (Bodner et al., 2020; Pickel et al., 2022).

In point of fact, describing this situation as paradoxical is inaccurate if we consider that past as well as more contemporary health, political, and economic crises (not to mention spectacular transportation catastrophes) have, as a rule, led to heightened production of conspiracy theories. This time the tendency bore an additional, negative consequence in the form of a more robust vaccine scepticism. For instance, a representative sampling of the Polish population in May 2021 showed that "one quarter of all Poles is decisively anti-vaccine, one quarter is decisively pro-vaccine (unaffected by any arguments against vaccines), and the remaining half is situated somewhere in between – they want to get vaccinated, but harbor doubts" (Pacewicz, 2021). By the summer of 2021, a massive, multifocal social movement against the national inoculation program and SARS-CoV-2-related restrictions had intensified in Poland. Moreover, this campaign was supported by some representatives of the nationalist-rightwing government and of radical right groups. In Poland, in contrast to many Western European countries, no restrictions on entering public places were introduced for nonvaccinated people. Likely underpinning that approach was recognition of societal resistance and/or a schism in the ruling coalition (Mierzyńska, 2021). Naturally, such a state of affairs would significantly (though indirectly) prolong the pandemic's duration; it also deepened the severity and scope of its more disastrous (including fatal) consequences.

Against this backdrop, not only did analysis of COVID-19 conspiracy theories gain hardy, practical meaning, but so did reflections upon the key features of conspiracy theories overall. This may lead to fresh insight into the sources as well as the possibilities for curbing the social impact of these theories. In turn, analysis of conspiracy theory traits gives impetus to comparisons of one's own conclusions with those evolving from other scholarly approaches to the problem.

This can also inspire endeavours to undertake a meta-reflection into methodical and systematic thinking about conspiracy theories.

Both of these topics – conspiracy theories themselves and (in a manner of speaking) the theories of conspiracy theories – will be investigated in terms of their communicative features; especially the rhetorical will be borne in mind. It behoves us to start with the latter, meta-theoretical motif because the repetitiveness of some characteristics in the vast majority of contemporary analyses into the causes and traits of these theories deserves attention. Furthermore, it is worth considering that here, in this ostensibly wholly abstract realm of analytical concepts, may lie the reasons why a stance supported by sound argumentation (and despite noble intentions) is ineffective in neutralizing conspiracy theories. Indeed, such a stance might sometimes act counter-effectively and contribute to a hardening of the position of believers.

Subsequent to that discussion, the focus will shift to the types, characteristics, and communicative aspects of conspiracy theories, taking into account (among others) those related to the global spread of COVID-19. A review of these issues might (or so it seems) provide answers to a question regarding the bases for the success of such theories across a wide range of social milieux. This could also unveil clues as to which "conspiratorial" rhetorical devices should be deconstructed in order to curb the momentum of these theories.

2. Theories of conspiracy theories: An attempt at meta-reflection[1]

Fascinating itself is the history of the means by which conspiracy theories are thematised and problematised. Nevertheless, the subject is so broad that a systematic analysis lies beyond the purview of this article.[2] From the standpoint taken herein, crucial is a shift in this very complex history, one that occurred after the Second World War. Prior to that war, conspiracy theories were often intertwined (it is worth emphasising) with openly declared antisemitic content. These took the form of notions involving some "Jewish conspiracy" and were widespread in mainstream public discourse across the European continent. The organization and execution of the Shoah on that same continent led to a postwar politics that mostly delegitimized antisemitic conspiracy theories which were

1 Other perspectives on meta-reflection are offered by Michał Otrocki (2007) and Franciszek Czech (2015).

2 One historical review depicting conspiracy theories in European culture can be found in Michael Butter and Peter Knight (2019). Cf. Butter 2020 (91–107) and Graumann & Moscovici 1987.

now seen as a component of precisely the mainstream discourse which had directly rationalised genocide. With that, conspiracy thinking, too, lost its overall societal legitimacy – yet this did not mean that it (including that antisemitic variant) vanished from the face of the Earth. Quite the contrary, they were and still are doing quite well in the domain of private communication and in that of radical political circles.

Noteworthy is that the expounding of antisemitic and racial prejudices has undergone a similar shift. Statements made in this vein ceased to be freely accepted in public and were even considered irrational. Still, something else happened which would bear consequences in the further evolutions of conspiracy theories. The very loss of antisemitism and racism's assumed obviousness – in addition to a legitimization pressure that would be adjunct to the propagation of socially unacceptable views – led to the development of new means by which prejudice could be communicated. Now one only needed to begin by declaring a rejection of prejudice as, indeed, irrational in order to continue relaying it, albeit in such a way as to evidence that one is nevertheless a rational human being. In practice this meant a kind of giftwrapping of antisemitic and racist statements with declared reservations (e.g., "I have nothing against Jews, but…") and attempts to justify one's reluctance towards Others (e.g., arguments recalling allegedly "objective" facts, illustrations of suitably interpreted anecdotal situations, etc.) (Billig, 1991, 122–141). Another important feature in the communication of prejudices is ascription to oneself of the "difficult job" of preaching an unwanted "truth."

There is a historical relationship between prejudice and the most radical, openly discriminatory, and ultimately criminal conspiracy theories. Due to that relationship, the postwar diffusion of the as-if rationalized prejudice pattern could not go without affecting the transformation of conspiracy theories. Under legitimization pressure, such theories began to reach increasingly for cherry-picked elements of scientific rhetoric. They would, for instance, gather information in support of a conspiracy view or almost routinely cite the authority of experts with academic degrees – albeit usually in a different field of knowledge than that pertaining to the conspiracy narrative. Finally, assigning themselves the purported function of disclosing an officially forbidden truth, conspiracy theories gained (in the eyes of their devotees) the valour of the righteously rebellious and unfairly excluded counter-knowledge.

Scholarly investigations into the phenomenon took place precisely in this context of postwar trends in the development of conspiracy theories. An important component of that context was a shift in the focus of social fears. As Butter (2020, 100) expressed this pithily: "In short, whereas we used to be afraid of conspiracies, we are now more afraid of conspiracy theories." A lesson stemming from World War II was that conspiracy theories should not only be ignored, but that the populace should be warned against their destructive potential, because reckless permission given for an unleashing of their capacity could lead to explosions of hatred and violence or, at the very least, to openly unjust, harmful practices and decisions.

Such consequences were further augmented by the emergence of new postwar conspiracy theories of a political sort – such as the search for evidence of a purported communist plot in America's artistic-intellectual milieux in the McCarthy era. An important voice on this subject was a book whose first edition appeared in 1956, *The Torment of Secrecy* written by a sociological luminary, Edward Shils (1996). More interestingly, Shils pointed not so much to the psychological as the ideological cornerstones for the "fear of conspiracy" of his time with its hyper-patriotism and radical populism. Reaching the West, along with the mid-1950s (so-called) "thaw" in the USSR and other countries of the "real socialism" bloc, was cognizance of the infamous role conspiracy theories had played in sustaining the Stalinist regime. By means of intimidation and torture, numerous individuals had been forced to confess to participation in nonexistent conspiracies; rigged trials led to many a death sentence.

Thus delegitimization and stigmatization of conspiracy theories became the permanent backdrop for analyses thereof. Testifying to this was the expression "paranoid style" in the title of a text by Richard Hofstadter (1966) – the most influential postwar text on this topic. Hofstadter patently and unequivocally emphasized that the word "paranoid" was not intended in a clinical, psychiatric sense. His aim in using that phrasing was to point to a unique mode of the political imagination, expressing itself via a certain way of communicating.[3] Although he wished to avoid psychiatric undertones, by the very fact of using such a label he inadvertently opened the door to precisely these connotations. Many commentators unwittingly picked up on the (misleading) psychiatric note, often lending an impression that they had not read beyond the title. Yet reading Hofstadter's text today, the original meaning still holds. Since the last decade of the 20th century (with evident intensification in the first decades of the 21st), a trend of research into conspiracy culture has been taking shape. It is in this context and looking retrospectively that Hofstadter's concept manifests itself as precursory.

3 The full title of his work was *The Paranoid Style in American Politics*. It is worth recounting this key (though often dismissed) statement in full: "I call it the paranoid style simply because no other word adequately evokes the qualities of heated exaggeration, suspiciousness, and conspiratorial fantasy that I have in mind. In using the expression 'paranoid style,' I am not speaking in a clinical sense, but borrowing a clinical term for other purposes. I have neither the competence nor the desire to classify any figures of the past or present as certifiable lunatics. [....] It is the use of paranoid modes of expression by more or less normal people that makes the phenomenon significant" (Hofstadter, 1966, 3–4).

Researchers in this subdiscipline signal a distance taken from the still common, dominant tendency toward a psychologising and pathologising of conspiracy theories. Among other aspects, researchers now turn their attention to 1) the cultural conditions for the popularity of conspiracy theories; 2) the fundamental components of a belief in such theories; 3) characteristics of conspiracy theories as attributes of a worldview; 4) conspiracy theories as a form of knowledge about reality; 5) patterns of communication in these theories (including narratives, modes of argumentation, and rhetorical features); 6) the role of conspiracy theories in political life; or 7) the place of conspiracy theories in pop culture.[4] Indubitably, the evolution of research into conspiracy culture favours a cultural turn (or turns) taking place simultaneously across the whole of the social sciences (Bachmann-Medick, 2016). Yet observation of the spread of conspiracy theories at the turn of the 20th and 21st centuries gives rise to certain impulses. Conspiracy theories have ceased to be a hallmark of the radical right or left; they have become very powerful in the cultural and political mainstream as well as in broader social (and internet) circles.

It is worth adding that, under the effects of this tendency, a misleading thesis is sometimes formulated that we are dealing today with a unidirectional process by which conspiracy theories expand. The result is an allegedly exceptional "age of conspiracy". As Joseph Uscinski and Joseph Parent (2014) showed – alongside evident political and cultural turning points – there have been waves of increased conspiracy theory popularity in Western culture. Hence, it would be more accurate to speak in the plural of the "ages of conspiracy" – one of which is nigh.

On the one hand, this cultural trend is developing intensively; on the other, there is further, rather extensive development of psychological research.[5] Interestingly, both trends – the cultural and psychological – are developing in parallel fashion, practically without communicating with one another. As a rule, psychological research does not make reference to cultural analyses. And yet cultural analyses do often critique the psychological approach – something that remains unnoticed by the other side.

Numerous are the psychological studies – both those presenting empirical research and those dealing with the theoretical concepts involved in conspiracy theories. However, the sheer quantity of psychological studies does not seem to go hand in hand with conceptual richness. Despite taking up various psycho-

4 Testifying to the significance of this cultural trend is that it can be found on the pages of the *Routledge Handbook of Conspiracy Theories* (Butter & Knight, 2020), as well as its strong presence in subsequent volumes of Routledge's *Conspiracy Theories* series (Harambam, 2020; Hristov, 2019; Madisson & Ventsel, 2021). Enlightening, too, is a comparison of the first and second editions of *A Culture of Conspiracy* by Michael Barkun (2003, 2013).

5 See, for instance, the review of the psychological research into conspiracy theories found in Pilch et al. 2023.

logical aspects, repeated in these texts are the same basic figures of thought that highlight the irrational nature of conspiracy theories and the irrational (or even paranoid) traits found in the psyches of their supporters. The far-reaching modelling of theories of conspiracy theories leads to an assumption that the theories about these theories are perhaps even more schematic than present-day conspiracy theories themselves. Contrary to appearances, the latter are, in fact, quite diverse (see the commentary on the variants below).

Two comments come to mind when looking at this tendency for psychological studies to proliferate while concurrently becoming more conceptually schematic. Firstly – in accord with the sociological concepts of Pierre Bourdieu (see 1991, 127), subsequently developed by Norman Fairclough (2013, 76ff) as an aspect of discourse analysis – whenever dealing with an overtly, universally accepted opinion or thesis, we should consider each time the role played by symbolic power. In other words, a lack of questioning of some point of view should not encourage singing with the choir that explicitly or implicitly affirms that stance. Quite the opposite, we should be even more bound to a seeking out of the social mechanisms that form and reinforce an unquestioned position. Bourdieu states that misrecognition of arbitrariness arises in such cases – e.g., an imperceptibility of the fact that a purportedly obvious truth has been socially shaped – alongside a simultaneous recognition of that truth's validity (Bourdieu & Wacquant, 1992: passim). In the footsteps of Bourdieu, Fairclough accents that the dominance of a certain discourse in a given social circle lies in the very fact that it goes unchallenged. Moreover, common sense is a product of that discourse type's naturalisation – meaning that this discourse is acknowledged as the natural way of speaking out on a given subject. As Fairclough (2012, 76) puts it, "naturalization is the royal road to common sense." Commonsensical theses that are binding in a given social context are not ideologically neutral.

Through this prism it is worth considering a widespread psychologisation, or even the psychiatrisation of conspiracy theories in psychological as well as everyday discourse; it is also worth looking into how psychological and everyday knowledge is impervious to other points of view, especially arguments stemming from studies into conspiracy culture. Psychological and everyday theories about conspiracy theories offer a representation according to which the propagation of or acquiescence to conspiracy theories not only wholly contradicts the rigours of scientific research but also goes beyond psychological normalcy. In other words, it is the domain of people incapable of rational thinking or, more colloquially, "crackpots". Key in this is that the conspiracy theories themselves are treated as an aberration – not because of some internal problems in their cultural milieu, but as a "foreign body" or "virus" that attacks the healthy tissue of mainstream culture from the outside.

A second observation is the abruptness with which the authors and supporters of psychological theories of conspiracy theories cut themselves off from conspiracy theories themselves. This is especially evident when, from the position of those representing science, such academics concentrate on the personalised discreditation of the propagators and devotees of conspiracy theories. Coming to mind here is a rhetorical question posed by Michel Foucault (2003, 10) with reference to "the aspiration to power that is inherent in the claim to being a science": "What types of knowledge are you trying to disqualify when you say that you are a science? What speaking subject, what discursive subject, what subject of experience and knowledge are you trying to minorize when you begin to say: 'I speak this discourse, I am speaking a scientific discourse, and I am a scientist.'"

That said, a crucial caution must be relayed. Foucault not only problematises science's aspirations to power over knowledge officially seen as insignificant – he goes even further. Contesting sanctioned science's pretensions to the throne, Foucault backs (in an anarchising spirit) alternative forms of knowledge, not noticing differences among them and striving "to enable them to oppose and struggle against the coercion of a unitary, formal, and scientific theoretical discourse" (2003, 10).

On one side of the coin – keeping in mind the socially harmful wielding of deep prejudices and hurtful slander in conspiracy theories – that additional, affirmative move is, in my opinion, intellectually and morally unacceptable. It does not resolve the methodological refusal to take a position here on the veracity or the moral dimension of conspiracy theories as proposed in the radical type of conspiracy culture study (see, for instance, Harambam, 2020, 227–238). Yet not taking a stand vis-à-vis socially destructive statements implies permission for just such communicative acts.

Constituting the other side of the coin is the fact that some conspiracy theories (even those initially ridiculed) occasionally turn out to be true (or at least partially accurate). If taken seriously enough in advance, this could develop into something socially useful (see Dentith, 2018). It would thus appear that the disadvantages as well as potential advantages of conspiracy theories should be, in each case, consciously and carefully considered – without escaping to a top-down affirmation, condemnation, or a stance that is (at least on the surface) neutral.[6]

6 A multilateral consideration of the potential benefits of conspiracy theories is proposed by Douglas et al. (2019, 17). It is worth noting that the literature review by these authors is testimony to a widening of the lens in analyses of conspiracy theories. With regards to determinants, not only the psychological factor comes to the fore, but also the social, cultural, and political. Additionally, the authors analyse the ways conspiracy theories are communicated and their impact on social life.

Nevertheless, Foucault's critique of academia's pretensions to symbolic power does bear positive meaning: it is sensitive to the serious risks associated with the stigmatisation of the representatives of alternative knowledge. Concerning the issue under discussion here, what matters is that an academic psychologisation of the matter of conspiracy theories – leading to a stigmatisation of their propagators and supporters – might be more conducive to the consolidation of their belief in the accuracy of a conspiracy theory than to their distancing from such. Personal criticism of "crackpots" (in the context of everyday communication, too) is also met with something of a psychologically understandable resistance. Quite different is, however, an extremely necessary, (self)critical look at the often poisoned discourse surrounding conspiracy theories and the unique culture of conspiracy – albeit without defining that culture as one that is foreign, and with a readiness to accept a thesis that conspiracy culture originates in the cultural mainstream. If it is at all possible for some means of persuasion to weaken faith in conspiracy theories then, it would seem, that goal would only be reached thusly.

Here the situation is similar to social reactions to prejudices which (after all) conspiracy theories often put to use. Years ago Margaret Wetherell and Jonathan Potter warned against the discursive strategy of "splitting" which – in the context of racism – comprises a unequivocal separation of the prejudiced from the nonprejudiced, self-identification with nonprejudiced folk, and a sort of externalisation of biases beyond one's own social circle (see, for instance, Boromisza-Habashi, 2015, 9). Along these lines, "a bestial other can be constructed who is different from self. The other is presented as driven by 'id-type' forces of irrational emotion and illogical dislike. While the self, in contrast, becomes all ego – a rational, thoughtful and reflective subject who speaks with the authority of facts" (Wetherell & Potter, 1992, 214). An analogous problem involves reactions to hate speech and conspiracy theories. Although a critical approach to tainted language is, for many reasons, advisable, the strategy of splitting (and, by the same token, conferring upon oneself a discursive innocence) is not only irrelevant, but also counter-effective as a means by which to battle and offset hate speech or conspiracy theories.

Standard, psychological, and commonsensical approaches do apply splitting against promoters and fans of conspiracy theories – and thus symbolically exclude these persons from the milieu of what is culturally binding. Along the way, such approaches hinder access to a distanced and critical look at the genesis of the conspiracy theories. A less straightforward path to a hypothetical reconstruction of those origins would, among others, wend its way by considering the communicative functions that conspiracy theories fulfil. In all certainty, conspiracy theories propose a picture of the world that is free of chance and unintended consequences – a world that is consistent and coherent. Therefore, one could say that conspiracy theories (despite appearances) are a response to the need for a rational image of the world. Common sense – which, in this case, is not the best advisor – fallaciously submits that the events and phenomena around us cannot be the result of reactions by anonymous social or cultural factors, but are, rather, the result of the realised, ignominious intentions of people acting in accord with those very intentions. Yet if it comes to unfavourable and chaotic events and phenomena, then the harmonisation of the overall image must lead to the imagining of certain causative entities guided (in some obscure way) by base motives. Hence, thanks to conspiracy theories, the world becomes (in the eyes of their supporters) clear anew. Solid support for this psychosocial mechanism is provided by long-term cultural change.

At this point, it is worth perusing the conclusions of the so-called sociological institutionalism. Social scientists from this circle proclaim the increasing importance of the cultural idea of agency in Western civilisation and (due to globalisation) around the world (see, for instance, Meyer & Jepperson, 2000). Old ways for translating reality – via reference to divine intervention, fate, the laws of nature, etc. – give way to explanations which point to the agency of individual and collective entities. In this context, probably justifiable is a thesis regarding "agency panic" as one of the factors conducive to the development of a contemporary culture of conspiracy. According to the author of this thesis, Timothy Melley (2002, 62), agency panic is anchored in an "intense anxiety about an apparent loss of autonomy or self-control – the conviction that one's actions are being controlled by someone else, that one has been 'constructed' by powerful external agents."

Nearly every researcher would likely agree that such psychosocial and cultural mechanisms could shape a proclivity to create conspiracy theories and succumb to them. Crucial, however, is that not everyone in this field goes on to also pose questions about the cultural sources of those mechanisms. Worth adding is that one of the conditions for unease and an unsatisfied need to feel that all is in order is the centuries-old tradition of European rationalism – already cultivated in ancient, classic philosophy, deepened in Enlightenment culture, and nurtured by contemporary academia – fostering that discomfort. Without reference points (i. e., rational patterns for interpretation of the surrounding world) impossible would be identification of circumstances perceived as irrational, and an immediately applied argumentation leading to the unleashing of rational principles that could guide the organisation of reality. However, unleashed in a pessimistic version of this process would be conspiracy theories. From this perspective, these theories are not a "foreign object" that fell on European lands, but are, instead, an inevitable side effect – a perverse, flip side of the coin of rationalist tradition. Underscored, too, should be that manifold are the circumstances in our times which (coupled with a latent expectation that the world, in principle, is in order) provide exceptionally strong impetuses for feelings that the world is becoming increasingly jumbled and muddled. Aside from obvious, shocking crisis situations (e.g., pandemics, wars, migration crises,[7] etc.), another contributing factor is the policy of diversity and the unpredictability of contemporary social reality. Stef Aupers (2019) points to three areas in which insecurity is rising, silently running in the background of daily routines: 1) epistemological insecurity is connected with a questioning of beliefs in the objectivity of science; 2) ontological insecurity refers to a general lack of certainty with regards to whether something is real or only staged; and 3) existential insecurity stems from the loss of certainty in one's worldview heretofore, leading to searches for new, ancillary pillars of support. All three of these are not so much the result of the hooking up of external factors to modernisation processes. Quite the contrary, the three realms are derived from the internal dynamics of modernisation processes – but at the same time they are fertile soil for the development of conspiracy culture.

The outline presented here of the standard scholarly (psychological) approach to conspiracy theories places in doubt the effectiveness with which such knowledge and analysis can face the task of neutralising such theories. Vast human experience thus far has indicated that this difficult task may not be feasible at all. Nonetheless, if an attempt at partial success were to be made, then science would need to meet at least the following preconditions: 1) dispense with the notion that academia is an unwavering bulwark of reason as well as a reliable provider of criteria for a lack thereof, and 2) cultivate the development of science without losing sight of a need for constant self-critical reflection upon assumed premises, research procedures, and the social functions that scholarship can fulfill.

3. Conspiracy theories and their variants

One could speak more precisely about a typology of conspiracy theories, if it were possible to determine what conspiracy theories are at all. Yet that issue is debatable. One resolution of this problem is proposed by Michael Barkun, according to whom virtually all conspiracy theories share three common elements, three fundamental components of their worldview:

- "*Nothing happens by accident.* Conspiracy implies a world based on intentionality, from which accident and coincidence have been removed. [….]

7 For more on the problematic nature of "migration crisis," see Krzysztof Jaskułowski (2019, 32ff) who points out that this term suggests that the problem lies with the migrants and not with others' reactions towards migration waves.

- *Nothing is as it seems.* Appearances are deceptive, because conspirators wish to deceive in order to disguise their identities or their activities. [....]
- *Everything is connected.* Because the conspiracists' world has no room for accident, pattern is believed to be everywhere, albeit hidden from plain view" (Barkun, 2013, 3–4).

Here, erring on the side of caution, Barkun's definition could be treated as referring to conspiracy theories in their model, radical and full meaning. This would leave the door open to considerations of such conspiracy theories which only partially meet the above-listed criteria. Therefore, for the purposes of the argumentation presented herein, conspiracy theories will be recognised as those imaginings which completely or partly match Barkun's benchmarks, even if identification of all the essential features requires further specification.

In widespread understandings of "conspiracy theory" – be they academic or colloquial – the term refers to agency by one or a small number of people who consciously (though secretly), and guided by base motives (e.g., hatred, lust for power, profit-seeking, etc.), act to the detriment of other persons or broader social groups. Recent tropes matching this paradigm include, for instance, COVID-19 conspiracy theories which tie the sources of the coronavirus itself and/or the mass vaccination campaigns to some underhanded motives of Bill Gates or George Soros as purportedly iconic representatives of a "world Jewry" aiming for global rule. Of course, this is not the only variant of conspiracy theories. One could point to a range of criteria by which variations differ from one another, which would bring us closer to a fuller depiction of what conspiracy theories are in general.[8]

The first category depends on the differentiation of classic versus network conspiracy theories. Described by the word "classic" are all of the just-mentioned ideas: hiding behind a façade of false explanations pertaining to unfortunate events lies the real truth about harmful activities taken by sinister social actors known by name, and those in complicity with them. The best known Polish case of such "classic" thinking is that concerning the 10 April 2010 airplane crash in which President Lech Kaczyński, his wife, and 94 others perished near Smoleńsk, Russia: the theory proclaims that, in reality, Russian President Vladimir Putin had colluded with the Polish then-Prime Minister Donald Tusk to bring down the plane.[9] Since the full, February 2022 Russian invasion of Ukraine – in tune with the disclosures of the scale and intensity of Russian war crimes – the so-called

8 Other typologies are proposed by Butter (2020, 14–18) and Anton & Schink (2021, 38–46).
9 Journalists of the liberal online medium, OKO.press (Pacewicz & Piechowicz, 2016) have described 24 varieties of this theory. Despite the differences, all the variations culminate in a thesis that President Kaczyński was murdered and that a search for this truth is a patriotic duty.

Smoleńsk conspiracy has again come to the fore in Polish mass discourse. However, it did not reappear as a result of new evidence proving the conspiracy theory, but rather in keeping with a typecast: "what the Russians are capable of."

In comparison, network conspiracy theories do not assign responsibility for crisis events or processes to concrete individuals, but rather to anonymous social networks. It was in line with such thinking that the pre-COVID-19 anti-vaxxer movement espied a pharmaceutical industry conspiracy in immunisation campaigns. Polish rightwing-nationalist media, in turn, see an unspecified "homolobby" conspiracy in the struggle for LGBTQ+ rights. More recently, COVID conspiracy theories have given rise not only to the earlier-described, classic variants, but network ones, too. The latter type has focused especially on an unspecified liberal elite that, under the banner of the Great Reset Initiative, was attempting to augment its financial and worldview advantages; that theory proclaims that the initiative was developed by liberals in a vast plot to depopulate the Earth, shape a novel type of human being, and create new social relations. It is true, however, that compared to Western European countries, the Great Reset Initiative network conspiracy theory is lesser known in Poland where (with respect to the coronavirus) classic theories dominate.[10]

The network type of conspiracy theories possesses a few persuasive advantages over the classic type: 1) there is no need to name specific persons (something that could be readily questioned) as conspiring perpetrators; 2) one can facilely link it to academic theses (widespread in social and political science, but also prevalent in pop culture and mass discourse) about the mounting role of social networks that encompass many areas of social life.[11] Another advantage of the network type is that propagators can, in their eyes, rebuff conspiracy thinking accusations by advocating the network concept of social life. By narrowing the scope of the conspiracy theory notion to its classic, personalised, and intellectually unsophisticated variant, they can (not without a bit of derisive irony) declare that the conspiracy thinking label does not apply to them. Moreover, by

---

10 Nevertheless, see, for instance, texts in Poland presenting and popularizing the Great Reset conspiracy theory such as *Wielki Reset* (2021).

11 Testimony to the diffusion of the concept of a network organization of social life is the book, *The Square and the Tower* by the popular historian, Niall Ferguson (2017). Although this volume abounds in controversial theses and far-reaching simplifications (e.g., the author's premise that a departure from hierarchies in favour of networks, despite certain advantages, will incur a fundamentally negative impact on social organization), it is impossible not to agree with two of Ferguson's observations. Firstly, social networks can tend to be conspiratorial (e.g., the organized attack on the World Trade Center on 11 September 2001), though there is no shortage of conspiracies in hierarchical societies. Secondly, in network as opposed to hierarchical social structures, there is no systematic documentation, no paper trail – something that can lead to a network's being perceived as the foundation for potential conspiracies.

emphasising the network nature of the effects of purportedly destructive ideas and behavioural patterns, network conspiracy promulgators apply only the intellectually ambitious (and generally recognised as valid) concepts of the network social order as developed precisely in social and political science.

The ambiguousness surrounding network conspiracy theories opens the door to semantic manipulation. In 2023, new information was published in Polish media indicating that Archbishop Cardinal Karol Wojtyła (later Pope John Paul II) had covered up cases of paedophilia among subordinate clergy. In response to these reports, a political and media front in defence of John Paul II was formed, one of whose slogans was that the disclosure constituted a second[12] assassination attempt – referencing the events of 13 May 1981 on Saint Peter's Square in the Vatican. That actual attempt on the Pope's life was (in light of investigations) quite likely the effect of a real political conspiracy, even if the identities of its principals were never indisputably established. This "second attempt" tag in 2023 could be understood not only as a loose metaphor but also as a suggestion that publication of that information about Archbishop Wojtyła could be part of a camouflaged plot by some unidentified, collective campaign against the Roman Catholic Church.

Additional aspects of the relationship between classic and network conspiracy theories become evident when we consider three differences setting real conspiracies apart from false, theoretical ones: 1) "the timescale of the alleged plot," 2) the number of people involved, and 3) the relationship between intentions and the effects of actions undertaken. Plots in the real world usually come to fruition within a relatively brief period, involve a handful of persons or a small group, and the scheme has a concrete objective (such as an assassination) designated by the conspirators. In contrast, (presumably false) conspiracy theories entail activities of a long duration, incorporating large numbers of insiders who (seem to be) moving towards some broad strokes goals. These are seen to be occurring despite well-founded contemporary, social sciences knowledge that historical processes cannot be planned and especially collective action is generally accompanied by unintended, even unanticipated or rather unwanted consequences (Butter, 2020, 18–23).

On the one hand, this reasoning seems to argue that we should not discard network conspiracy theories as automatically incorrect, but rather treat them

12 This catchphrase was introduced into Polish public discourse by Archbishop Marek Jędraszewski, a successor to the same archdiocese of Kraków in which Karol Wojtyła had served. In Jędraszewski's sermon, delivered during the mass on 7 March 2023, he stated that responsible for this "second attempt" were "the same circles" who had been responsible for the first one on the pope. See https://diecezja.pl/aktualnosci/abp-marek-jedraszewski-o-drugim-zamachu-na-sw-jana-pawla-ii-jego-glos-jest-ciagle-glosem-sprzeciwu-dlatego-probuje-sie-go-zniszczyc/ (27 June 2023).

with some scepticism as potentially false. On the other hand, although classic conspiracy theories do tend to be fallacious, it would be wise to refrain from a blanket prejudgment because they may turn out to be true. Hence it appears that the common, almost routine identification of conspiracy theories with false representations of reality is not as obvious as might seem, and so another dividing line could be drawn between inaccurate and accurate conspiracy theories (the latter concerning real conspiracies).[13]

A still greater testing of the limits of the meaning of "conspiracy theory" are plots or actually collusions agreed to in good faith, with noble intentions – not to hinder, humiliate, or harm anyone, but rather to help and support someone. A fitting example here could be the collusive conspiracies in the medical and or familial contexts analysed by the sociologist, Erving Goffman (1971, 337–340). This type of "conspiracy" not only does occur, but is often routine practice in hospitals and at home. Yet this should not, in my opinion, lead to expansion of the concept of conspiracy theory to such an extent as to encompass benign collusion. Diluted along the way would be what, apparently, is a key determinant for conspiracy theories – that is, that they (accurately or inaccurately) refer to plots founded on disreputable motives.

A further criterion splits conspiracy theories into the bottom-up and the top-down. Grassroots conspiracy theories are created and spread by ordinary people – mainly via gossip and rumour in the past, now more often through the internet. Hierarchic conspiracy theories are initiated and disseminated by government agencies. The dividing line, however, is not a sharp one: the former are a tasty morsel for political actors who can instrumentalise these conspiracy theories for their own usage, whereas the latter are constructed to tug at the heartstrings of the popular imagination, finding favour in bigger social circles.

Coronavirus conspiracy theories have been, for the most part, of a grassroots nature. Their hallmark is an emphasis on questioning the authority of generally-accepted scientific findings as well as a clearly anti-elitist and, more generally, anti-establishment, polemical tone. The top-down conspiracy theories are transmitted via communication media (sometimes as part of a widescale propaganda campaign) and serve to increase political sway or to cement the position of the currently ruling political elite. Keeping all differences in mind, examples of such top-down conspiracy theories include ideas about spy rings which justified the so-called Great Purge of the Stalinist USSR, notions of a communist threat surfacing in the McCarthy era in the USA, or, quite contemporaneously, an imagined Western conspiracy targeting present-day Russia (the official rationalisation for Russia's 2022 full invasion of Ukraine). Of a network nature was the

13 It must be added here that Michael Butter (2020, 36–67) sees this differently, excluding the category of accurate conspiracy theories.

(criminal in its consequences) top-down III Reich vision with its extremely antisemitic, verbally and visually communicated image of an alleged Jewish conspiracy.

Particularly popular conspiracy theories are of both the top-down and bottom-up types. This pertains especially to situations in which a populist political leader presents him or herself as the representative of average folk, an opponent to the supposedly corrupt elites. A fusion of both these types, anchored in accusations of fake news as well as actual misinformation, assisted Donald Trump in gaining the presidency of the United States. A similar fusion of the two types shaped itself with respect to the Smoleńsk airplane catastrophe described earlier. In this case, too, top-down declarations by representatives of the government and the political party represented by the late President were met halfway by bottom-up statements made by bloggers and social media posts by average citizens. A key moment in this 2010 conspiracy theory's evolution was a 2022 statement by Jarosław Kaczyński (the deceased president's twin brother as well as leader of the then ruling *Prawo i Sprawiedliwość* party): on the 12th anniversary of the crash, Kaczyński proclaimed publicly that Vladimir Putin was responsible for the catastrophe thus turning a conspiracy theory into an official "truth" confirmed by the government.[14] However, according to representative sample surveys, popular support for this version remains at about one-third of the adult population.[15] This confirms a thesis formulated by Michael Butter (2022, 11) in the foreword to the Polish translation of his book: in Poland and the USA (as opposed to Germany) it happens that conspiracy theories are advocated by representatives of the political leadership, becoming not only a heterodox anti-knowledge, but also an orthodox official knowledge.

Apart from the top-down and bottom-up categories, it is prudent to also differentiate between central and peripheral conspiracy theories: those in which the main roles are played by the political and economic elite, influential individuals, and others holding high status in the social structure vis-à-vis those whose conspirators are found at lower levels of the social structure. Key in this case are not the top-down and bottom-up conspiracy theories themselves, but how those theories are envisioned and the impressions they make. Yet another categorisation appears when the criterion is whether conspirators are insiders, belonging to the social milieu which a conspiracy theory concerns, or are (perceived as) outsiders to that milieu. In other words, the focus is on conceptions that see a conspiracy as internal or external to the group.

14 See the interview with Jarosław Kaczyński for the weekly, *Sieci* No 14/2022, 4–10.04.2022, 11.

15 According to a survey published in April 2023, even 38% of the Polish population believes that the "Smoleńsk catastrophe" could be the result of an assassination ordered by Vladimir Putin; see https://www.pap.pl/aktualnosci/news%2C1563823%2Csondaz-ilu-polakow-wierzy-ze-w-smolensku-byl-zamach.html (22 April 2023).

As mentioned earlier, the accuracy-inaccuracy divide should also be taken under consideration. A natural question, however, is whether accurate conspiracy theories should be described using the same terminology as those theories which are blatantly false and ofttimes based on xenophobia. The decision here to apply "conspiracy theory" to both these variations is connected, on the one hand, with a distancing from the psychological pathologisation of conspiracy theories. On the other hand, we should not forget that history as well as the present have provided much evidence to the effect that correct or partially correct ideas on the topic of actual plots tend first to be discredited as false conspiracy theories – only to (with time) gain social acknowledgement as true accounts. This reflection leads to a further classification divide between conspiracy theories which are socially accepted and those wholly unaccepted. Quite convincing might be arguments in favour of combining these two criteria – (in)accurate and (un)accepted – delineating four variants of conspiracy theories (see Anton & Schink, 2021, 43–46).

It should be accented that ambiguity is also characteristic of conspiracy theories as a sociological phenomenon. The fundamental understanding of this term implies a hyperbolic seeking out of conspiracies where they likely do not exist – and yet conspiracy culture can be the genuine reality. Literary illustrations of such a state of affairs have been provided by, among others, Honoré de Balzac in the second part of *The Lost Illusions.* He describes therein the "Parisian Machiavellianism" reigning among the journalistic-artistic circles of the French capital in his time – meaning numerous, small, ad hoc, and not thoroughly planned intrigues, tricks, and societal tactics whose aim it was to serve injury upon fellow participants in the same social circles (Balzac, 2004). Of course, insider knowledge about such practices could not help but exact watchfulness and wariness: constant was the risk of falling into a trap which, inevitably, led to an oversensitivity to that very possibility. In such situations a real "conspiracy culture" gives rise to a generalised, commonplace understanding of that term. In that latter sense, conspiracy culture might not be rooted in any reality or might be rooted in one only to a certain extent – depending upon the degree to which an atmosphere of heightened caution against potential conspiracies befits the real danger.

Summarising this section, the indistinctness of "conspiracy" opens the way to that word's heuristically-valued ambiguity as an attribute in the terms "conspiracy theory" or "conspiracy culture." Emerging from the combination of the first two criteria discussed are four variants of conspiracy theories: the classic bottom-up and top-down theories and the bottom-up and top-down network conspiracy theories. This set of variations begins to increase when we consider that each of the four can be more central or peripheral, more external or internal, more accurate or inaccurate, and socially accepted or unaccepted. Still, this raises a number of further questions about differences and similarities, as well as the possible connections between variants of conspiracy theories and culture. But these questions require a separate analysis. Overall, coming into view from the above-sketched outline of possible types of conspiracy theories is a richer picture of what conspiracy theories are as a whole.

4. Communicative aspects of conspiracy theories

Accountability and its complexities

"Accountability is a key ethnomethodological term (Garfinkel, 1967, 1ff) and refers to a constant process of producing verbal and non-verbal indications which the participants of a situation give to themselves and to each other to make 'observable -and-reportable' how they interpret their own and others' activities. Importantly, these interpretive indications are performed in and through these very activities" (Czyżewski, 2023, 33). Hence, ethnomethodology is interested in a, so to speak, self-oriented accountability of practical actions. For instance, an ethnomethodological conversation analysis studies, among other things, the way in which participants signal to each other – in and through their remarks – that they are in a pre-closing sequence which can lead to a mutually agreed-upon end to their conversation, though both are also open to continuance. A note to be added here is that research interests in ethnomethodology are focused on interpretive aspects of routine, often seemingly banal, everyday activities. By the same token, ethnomethodology offers a reanalysis of interpretive processes which first unfold in and through those activities themselves. In contrast to the ethnomethodological perspective, at the centre of the commentary presented herein is other-oriented accountability which refers to assorted aspects of reality, attempting to interpret them through various kinds of accounts (e. g., comments, reports, explanations, etc.).

Two circumstances appear to have especially intensively contributed to the fact that we do not simply live as distinct and separate individuals immersed in one and the same reality, but in collectively interpreted, varied realities. In other words, people do not possess their very own, individual access to reality, but are found in different, collectively-created interpretive cocoons. Firstly, vigorously expanding is the process of professional, quasi-professional, or utterly amateur production and dissemination of texts. The driving forces behind this inflationary production of texts are three primary "factories" generating interpretation: institutionalised science and higher education, mass media journalism, and amateur internet activity. Moreover, the boundaries between these three are not always impermeable.

Secondly, a clearly unsatisfied hunger for accounts succumbs to far-reaching amplification in situations perceived as particularly difficult, dangerous, or unexpected – such as an economic depression, war or pandemic. It is no wonder that all three "factories" feel called to confront such challenges and are ready to cover the excess, urgent need for interpretations. Naturally, in this context, too, demand can drive supply. New descriptions and narrations become the object of other-oriented meta-accountability if they are commented upon as especially accurate and helpful or as problematic, invalid, and unacceptable. In this way, the process of interpretation can get tangled in its own cocoon.

Here an idea comes to mind: at least some conspiracy theories could share much in common with science. In the context discussed here, what matters is that both these endeavours (i.e., conspiracy theories and science) strive to deliver socially-binding truths about reality – even if they employ different procedures and attain different results. A claim to be pronouncing the truth is particularly important when decisions of a political nature are legitimised by knowledge as an authority – and this is the situation in contemporary, modernised societies. As Alexander Bogner noted, an epistemisation of the political then occurs, a conflict over better knowledge becomes a camouflaged social and political conflict, and a "revolt of the ignorant" against the power of official knowledge is a consequence (Bogner, 2021).

Functions of this sort are fulfilled by, among others, grassroots conspiracy theories which are positioned as an alternative to science. The situation is somewhat different with the "top-down" conspiracy theories which are instrumentally constructed, purposely false, and disseminated through media of official indoctrination. Examples of such conspiracy theories in action have been the III Reich's antisemitism campaigns, Stalinist campaigns against alleged enemies of the regime during the Great Purge, or Russia's current anti-Ukrainian and anti-Western propaganda. Hierarchical conspiracy theories serve to cement the potentially absolute power of a political elite, challenged and contested by local intellectual elites only if they are prepared to take existential risks. Bottom-up conspiracy theories, in contrast, rebel not only vis-à-vis the political elite, but also the entire establishment, including its academic arm. These theories are commonly false, though their supporters wholly and passionately believe in them. Interestingly enough, when even one of these conspiracy theories does happen to be partially accurate, the conspiratorial style in which it is expressed becomes a pretext to reject all as ostensibly untrue, stigmatised as an aberration. The third variation comprises an alliance of top-down and bottom-up conspiracy theories – an iconic example of which is Donald Trump who is a representative of the political and economic elite, but has positioned himself as anti-elite and populist.

External and internal schemes of interpretation

In order to render specific phenomena (e.g., situations, events, actions, statements, etc.) accountable – via a conspiracy theory, for instance – appropriate symbolic resources need to be mobilised. Such resources offer a range of socially created, easily recognised, and conceptually generalised schemes of interpretation. Thanks to their application (often adapted to a concrete case) possible become a pre-classification and the assignment of specific features to a phenomenon requiring interpretation.

Interesting is the contrast emerging between various schemes of interpretation through which grassroots conspiracy theories are made accountable. Recapitulated first will be how bottom-up conspiracy theories are presented from an external viewpoint – in other words, what schemes of interpretation external to these theories in particular are applied to them. Meaningful here, too, is the widespread and degrading psychologization of all conspiracy theories (including the bottom-up). Ascribed to propagators and backers of conspiracy theories are at least two intellectual deficits, both constituting different aspects of a contention that these theories are unempirical.

Firstly, backers of conspiracy theories are denied a readiness and ability to confront the facts. The routine retort, "either something is a fact, or it's not" corresponds with a methodological postulate regarding the basic susceptibility of academic findings to falsification. At this point, the commonsensical maxim and the normative principle of a scholarly course of action mutually support each other. But not always is that normative principle accompanied by a self-critical constatation that, in fact, practice every so often strays from principle. As Ludwik Fleck (1981) accented in his sociology of science texts, academic group-think displays a sweeping tenacity; collective styles of thinking are, to a great degree, resistant to alternative standpoints and empirically demonstrated counterexamples.

Secondly, those who advocate and disseminate conspiracy theories are subjected to a symbolic psychiatrisation by way of stigmatising names such as "crackpot" or "madman." The temptation to employ such epithets is problematic for two reasons. On the one hand, the names are inapt as they label people who may be rightly concerned about conflicting information and are far from conspiracy views. On the other hand, personified stigmatisation is usually counterproductive since this can unintentionally contribute to the hardening of a heretofore latent conspiracy theory mindset. Here, too, common sense and a scientific mindset reinforce each other, although in an ill-fated covenant: the common sense assessment of "they're crazy" matches a political science reading that this is "political paranoia".

Internal schemes of interpretation – i. e., those applied to grassroots conspiracy theories by their propagator-backers – decidedly differ from external ones. A reliable reconstruction of the ways these schemes are utilised would necessitate a systematic analysis of specific statements (albeit beyond the purview of this text). However, to put it briefly, certain dimensions of internal schemes of interpretation can be isolated and identified which, in certain cases, are used in conjunction with one another:

- The dimension of power – freedom versus oppression. Bottom-up conspiracy theories are an expression of rebellion against and aim to liberate the people from the establishment;
- The horizontal dimension – periphery versus centre. Grassroots theories express the rebellion of the cultural, social, political, and economic peripheries against the cultural, social, political, and economic core. This refers to peripheral conspiracy theories although central ones also position themselves as a rebellion against some other core (e. g., presumably influential, external entities);
- The vertical dimension – a reversed classism. Since classism entails higher social classes looking down on lower ones with superiority and contempt, then reversed classism entails the lower classes looking on the higher ones with the undisguised rage of the healthy folk against the corrupt elites. It should be added that traditional and reversed classism are, as schemes of interpretation, capable of confirming the real class hierarchy, but can also define class differences. Regardless of the actual place that the authors and addressees of external schemes of interpretation occupy in the social structure, their declarations are accompanied by connotations of class superiority and contempt regarding the promotors and backers of conspiracy theories. In turn, the supporters of grassroots conspiracy theories emboss their statements on the subject of alleged conspiracists with a note of anger typical of reversed classism. Even if they belong to the upper levels of society with respect to wealth, prestige or popularity, they don the costumes of representatives of the common people, bringing enlightenment and emancipation;
- The moral dimension – good versus evil. Though it is clear from an external perspective that numerous conspiracy theories (including the grassroots) are infected by strong prejudices, the internal perspective leads to a completely different stance with regards to values. The image of reality is here presented by an abstract battle between good and evil in which propagators and supporters of conspiracy theories position themselves as heroic defenders of good against evil; and
- The dimension of demystification – truth versus lies. According to internal schemes of interpretation, the mission of (especially bottom-up) conspiracy

theories is a heroic telling of uncomfortable truths and opposition to the imposed, official falsehoods.

Three things come to mind here. Firstly, reviewing external schemes of interpretation, it is difficult to avoid a question about the extent to which the cultural and political establishment's lack of self-criticism could have contributed to the development of grassroots, anti system-oriented conspiracy theories. Secondly, turning attention to the internal schemes dampens the psychologisation of conspiracy theories and encourages an addressing of conspiratorial culture (whose reconstruction must be accompanied by its critique). Thirdly, communication practices that rely on polemical (accurate or inaccurate) attribution of the expounding or acceptance of conspiracy theories need to be distinguished from the external and internal schemes. The use of such attributions aims to discredit an adversary in a political or media dispute – a point to which I return in the conclusion, pointing to an interpretive approach to conspiracy theories.

Conspiracy theories and academia

Taken for granted is a premise according to which conspiracy theories constitute the contradiction of science and logic. In fact, a descriptor coming first to mind is that they are unscientific. That being concurrently a habitual accusation and a symbolic degradation of conspiratorial types of knowledge about the real world, it is not uncommon for reflections on the relationship between conspiracy theories and science to end here. Still, without questioning their unempirical nature, it is worth delving into the complex relations between such theories and academia. It is also worth considering whether the charge of an unscientific nature in conspiracy theories is useful in neutralising their persuasive power.

The first misgivings arise when taking into account contemporary, philosophical and sociological thinking about the status of empirical cognition – reflections pointing to the limited, historical, revocable, and socially-conditioned nature of that cognition. Paradoxically, it is surely conspiracy theories which have now usurped (exclusively) a claim to objective and impartial knowledge. In such a situation, that charge of irrationality (albeit accurate) is unconvincing for members of a conspiratorial culture, inasmuch as that accusation goes unsupported by supplementary argumentation.

Secondly, conspiracy theories make extensive use of academia's stylistic accessories. Richard Hofstadter (1966, 37) already called attention to this, ascribing a "striving for scholarly depth and an inclusive world" solely to a segment of the political spectrum: "The entire right-wing movement of our time is a parade of experts, study groups, monographs, footnotes, and bibliographies." It appears that this tendency is characteristic of present-day conspiratorial culture as a whole, regardless of political orientation, and yet Hofstadter (1966, 37) correctly highlights that the frailty in conspiracy theories lies elsewhere: "What distinguishes the paranoid style is not, then, the absence of verifiable facts (though it is occasionally true that in his extravagant passion for facts the paranoid occasionally manufactures them), but rather the curious leap in imagination that is always made at some critical point in the recital of events." Noteworthy in the accusation that conspiracy theories are unscientific is that "leap in imagination" – that is, drawing unfounded conspiratorial conclusions from an ofttimes correct and methodically developed diagnosis of a state of affairs.

Still, in discussion with a conspiracy theorist, it would not seem that an always effective argumentation would be what common sense first suggests as the right strategy, i.e., proven facts. On this subject, conspiracy culture participants usually have an opinion not subject to revision based on partially true knowledge of many a specific fact. It is prudent to consider that the scientificisation of modern conspiracy theories is part of a broader social process which Karl Mannheim (1956) referred to as "the democratization of culture." What Mannheim had in mind was, above all, a questioning and shortening of the distances between high and low (or popular) culture, between a work of art and its audience (whereby the work ceases to be an object of worship), and between a creator and their audience (whereby the artist is deprived of their aura of exceptionality) (Mannheim, 1956, 220–229; cf. Czyżewski, 2018). These same democratisation tendencies are evident today with reference to science.

Especially within a conspiracy culture, amateur, quasi-scientific activity is not only nurtured, but also placed on par with or above professional scholarship. At the same time, however, the average consumer (especially members of conspiracy cultures) can treat academic publications today without obligatory respect. These are, after all, one of many possible sources of information and their talking-head authors appear in the media on an equal level as other providers of reality interpretation. Instructive in this context is Mannheim's thesis that one of the components in the democratization of culture is a reevaluation in the area of how knowledge is formed. In this sense, democratisation means a "shift from the morphological to the analytical outlook" (Mannheim, 1956, 214). Morphological thinking explains the world in categories unanalysed as a whole, but experienced via symbols. In turn, the analytical approach breaks an object of cognition down into functional elements, asking about its structure, conditions, and consequences. As part of the democratisation process, the analytical perspective spreads throughout broad social circles; utilisation of that perspective becomes a sign of claims to the status of a full-fledged insider of the social order. Especially power is somewhat brought down to Earth: even if it is still an object of collective rituals, it is also increasingly the subject of disillusioned analyses (Mannheim

1956, 213–219). Thus, democratisation in the realm of knowledge is conducive to anyone and everyone becoming endowed with the chance to be a researcher of reality – just as a democratisation of the fine arts makes something of an artist of anyone.

Amateur quasi-scientific activity is, therefore, not some strange aberration deviating far from the direction taken by dominant cultural changes; it belongs to the mainstream (although indubitably harmful), if it serves to justify conspiracy theories. Furthermore, knowledge gaps or errors appearing in official, scientific versions of events do nothing to weaken trust in conspiracy theories. According to the classic concept of biased assimilation, a strong, a priori belief with regards to some issue (such as the accuracy of a given conspiracy theory) leads to unreserved acceptance of expert studies that support one's own view – even if there are disparities there as well. Consequently, expert studies contradicting one's own views are treated with singular inquisitiveness, a fervent seeking out of actual gaps and errors therein (Lord, Ross & Lepper, 1979).[16] Hence, not only does well-intentioned scholarly learning not have to lead to an intended goal, but may have the opposite effect: hardening a position which others wish to take apart, further exacerbating polarisation of attitudes. Naturally, circumstances can be more difficult when conspiracy theory supporters make use of disinformation and fake news. Unlike it was in Hofstadter's time, disinformation is now quite often the case. Although fake news call for corrections (e.g., through a questioning of their sources), achieving that goal can be difficult, if not impossible.

Thirdly and finally, a bandying about the unscientific tag can come too easily. Contemporary social reality provides many reasons to doubt its official political interpretations and give credence to conspiracy theories. For instance, made public are successive scandals connected with supra-legal, longstanding blockages of the justice system by powerful chemical corporations responsible for the acute illnesses and deaths of residents inhabiting areas contaminated due to the business activities of those corporations. Still more publicity has accompanied the disclosure of illegal surveillance of citizens via the latest, hard-to-detect information technologies. A serious challenge for contemporary Western societies is also the issue of overpopulation: the increasing numbers of people whose work is no longer needed and who therefore cannot afford the role of consumers. Such persons are the "unintended and unplanned 'collateral casualties' of economic progress" (Bauman, 2017, 39).

16 Lars Weisbrod (2022) discussed the biased assimilation concept, sceptically considering the effectivity of typical academic studies with reference to anti-vaxxers who became advocates of COVID-19 conspiracy theories.

These and a range of other reasons could lead many people to fundamental doubts about the transparently just social order of liberal democracy. Naturally, those reasons do not justify Hofstadter's "leap in imagination," steering the way from a partially accurate diagnosis to an unsubstantiated, conspiratorial conclusion. They do, however, merit the reporting of doubts that should not be automatically pigeonholed as manifestations of conspiracy thinking. After all, for many years there has been an ongoing, serious discussion on the crisis of liberal democracy and the sources of a new wave of populism in Western societies. Attention in this discussion is called to the difference between promises of freedom, equal opportunity, and prosperity (part and parcel of the liberal script) and the reality in which various kinds of deficits, abuses, and distortions bourgeon.

Yet it is a long way from this debate to belief in the Great Reset Initiative conspiracy. It is one thing to critically reflect upon the condition of liberal democracy, but quite another to instrumentally employ reservations about the liberal script in order to validate conspiracy theories. For example, Marek A. Zamorski (2020, 15–23) points to five present-day "myths that prevent us from understanding the world": "democracy as rule by the people," "free media," "the free market," "the objectivity of science," and "sovereign nation states". The problem lies in the fact that Zamorski treats these ideas as propaganda deceits intended to obscure the hidden schemes hatched by elites aiming to enlarge their power and wealth at the expense of a naïve citizenry. In accord with this thinking, the final stage in a longstanding, global conspiracy by the liberal elites is to be Operation Pandemic. Moreover, it is one thing to pose questions out of uncertainty and a desire to learn, and quite another to disgorge extensive sermons overflowing with conspiratorial insinuations, brought to a close by an ostensibly harmless, "I'm just asking."

Thus it is not worth airing conspiracy thinking where it does not yet exist. Nevertheless, it is worth agreeing with those who raise doubts about the condition of liberal democracy and the quality of its institutions; it is worth treating serious questions with respect. That said, however, concessions regarding a diagnosis should be accompanied by disagreement with conclusions that stem not from logical inference, but from a "leap in imagination".

A brief outline of conspiratorial rhetoric: The case of COVID-19 conspiracy theories

When conspiracy culture is viewed as a bundle of communication patterns, and not as a system of norms and values, then a key research question comes to mind: by what means of communication are conspiracy theories propagated and transmitted? A further question arises as to which methodological approach is best utilised, with one option being a research trend that investigates the interdependence between conspiracy narratives utilised in popular culture and conspiracy theories themselves (see Boltanski, 2014; Carver, Craciun & Hristov, 2020). Another path is discourse analysis which is what Jack Bratich (2008) employed in his description of the discourse of conspiracy panics.

With this in mind, outlined below will be an attempt to apply rhetorical analysis. This choice is connected with an assumption that the success of conspiracy theories may be a consequence of their communicative effectiveness (i. e., their persuasive power). That this may be the case is evidenced by the routinely raised and ritualised charge that conspiracy theories are unscientific – which does not, as a rule, convince supporters, but, in fact, further confirms their belief in the entanglement of official research studies in conspiracies. This subsequently means that efforts to counter conspiracy theories are in need of review.

Earlier herein there was talk of self-oriented and other-oriented accountability. The rhetorical aspects of conspiracy theories refer to yet a third kind of accountability which, like the latter of the first two, reaches beyond ethnomethodological interests.[17] This time, the point is that the meaning of a single utterance, text or conversation can sometimes go far beyond its local context, shaping the image of social life on a macro scale and sometimes social reality itself. One example of this is Martin Luther King's famous "I have a dream" phrase: on the one hand, a fragment of a specific speech, but, on the other hand, a commanding symbol of a collective political mobilisation.

Helpful in the reconstruction of rhetorical aspects of conspiracy theories can be one of the approaches found in rhetorical criticism today. This role can be fulfilled by Fantasy Theme Analysis (FTA) which deals with the dynamic processes of shaping an image of reality that is both convergent and symbolically resonant. Along this path, individuals are able to shape among themselves a community of ideas about reality, simultaneously signalling to each other that they belong to a community of human beings who share the same rhetorical vision. It should be accented that such a vision need not be false. What distinguishes rhetorical visions from ordinary pictures of reality is that the former arise and are maintained in the course of a particularly intense, mutual stimulation and winding up – something that Ernst Bormann, the creator of FTA, called chaining (Bormann, 1984; Foss, 2018). Noteworthy is Hofstadter's underscoring of the fact that conspiracy theory communication is often accompanied by "heated exaggeration, suspiciousness, and conspiratorial fantasy" (Hofstadter, 1966, 3). It appears that FTA terminology and especially the word "chaining"

17 For more on the subject of the three types of accountability, see Czyżewski, 2023.

(while avoiding the exaggerated psychiatric connotations of "paranoid style") describe exactly the phenomenon that Hofstadter had in mind.

Obviously, conspiracy theories constitute but one of the types of rhetorical visions. Still, this does not change the fact that, using the basic analytical categories of FTA, the recurring rhetorical characteristics of SARS-CoV-2 conspiracy theories can be identified and organised.

- ***symbolic triggers***
- ***fantasy themes***
- ***fantasy types***
- ***basic rhetorics***
- ***symbolic personae***

RHETORICAL VISIONS

Fig. 1: Analytical framework of FTA

Symbolic triggers

Sufficient as an impetus for a forceful and tightly focused conversation to develop is some evocative word or formulaic phrase bearing a recognisable connotation ("With that vaccine, it's hard to tell" or "Well, and all those restrictions").

Fantasy themes

The communicative exchange focuses on a single thematic field (here the coronavirus pandemic) which is treated by interlocutors as biographically and politically relevant.

Fantasy types

In the course of a conversation, emblematic stories are recounted (e.g., that hospitalized patients are not sick with SARS or that vaccines are harmful), with anecdotal illustrations allegedly proving the purported truth therein. Prompted often is a sequence of stories – i.e., a story told by one person inspires another participant in the conversation to narrate a similar tale.

Basic rhetoric

(Classic) conspiracy theories are supported by archetypical schemes of argumentation according to which standing behind all negative phenomena (e.g., allegedly false theses about the spread of the virus, the mass vaccination campaign, and the epidemiological restrictions) are egotistically-minded, powerful actors who (guided by base economic and political motives) manipulate public opinion and the general social reality.

Symbolic personae

Especially influential agency is credited to select, universally recognisable figures in economic or political life who are hypothetically responsible for all negative singularities associated with a conspiracy theory. With respect to the COVID-era conspiracy theories, the role of those with destructive, almost diabolical agency was assigned to Bill Gates and/or George Soros.

Rhetorical visions

Rhetorical visions can pertain to various issues. They can be positive (e.g., when celebrating the achievements of national heroes), or decidedly negative (e.g., when conspiracy theories arise). Either way, the rhetorical vision combines the above-mentioned components into a single whole, fulfilling the function of a worldview. A conspiratorial rhetorical vision proclaims that nothing happens by accident, without a reason. Reality, however, is not subject to anonymous rules and mechanisms, but shaped by ominous conspiracies. It is as a consequence of the conspiracies that all components of reality are expected to fit the puzzle, creating a seemingly coherent and incontrovertible picture. There is no room here for inconsistencies, but, if they should appear, then a conspiracy theory will easily prove that they are superficial.

5. On a third way

Apart from the two fundamental research approaches – the psychological and the cultural – it is worth pointing out the third, interpretive approach which, for the time being, remains (to a great extent) an open, but unrealised opportunity.[18] This time it would be, on the one hand, about an analysis of the ways in which dialogue partners, especially in public communication, accuse each other of participating in a conspiratorial pact; but, on the other hand, they attribute to each other the propagation of conspiracy theories or a belief in their accuracy.[19] This sort of looping of public communication often takes place in a polarised

18 See an interesting attempt by Jerzy Stachowiak (2023).

19 A divide into the psychological, cultural, and interpretive corresponds with the three sociologies: the first pertains to objective regularities, the second deals with cultural rules, and the third entails the methods of interpretation (see Eglin, 1978).

public sphere and actually determines its further polarisation. An additional factor reinforcing this tendency are, of course, election campaigns.

It is worth noting that the radical version of the interpretive approach is decidedly anti-psychological in character, and as such furnishes valid arguments against the psychologising of conspiracy theories. However, ethnomethodological and conversation analytic sources of skepsis toward psychological reasoning are not always acknowledged. In one of his early texts, Harold Garfinkel, the "father" of ethnomethodology, remarked that "I shall exercise a theorist's preference and say that meaningful events are entirely and exclusively events in a person's behavioural environment [...]. Hence there is no reason to look under the skull since nothing of interest is to be found there but brains. [...] Instead questions will be confined to the operations that can be performed upon events that are 'scenic' to the person" (Garfinkel 1963: 190). The continuators of ethnomethodological conversation analysis oppose the "cognitivist or mentalist preconceptions" which dominate social sciences, whereby an individual is thought of as "the bearer or container of the referents of the 'mental' vocabulary" (Watson & Coulter, 2008, 12). Apparently, the proponents of the psychological approach to conspiracy theories see the authors and supporters of such theories precisely in these terms, as evidenced by Watson and Coulter's further observations:

> Casual powers are attributed to several of these 'mental concepts' (e.g. 'motive', 'mental intention', 'mental interpretation') by various theorists [...]. Each and every one of these postulates is the result of treating our 'mental' vocabulary as if it consisted of labels for unobservable, inner phenomena and of treating what are occasioned and normative *practices* (e.g. 'interpreting', 'anticipating', 'monitoring') as if they were, instead, interior operations or processes to be analysed without reference to, or with only thin reference to, their particular occasioning context. (ibid., 12–13; cf. Czyżewski, 1989)[20]

Clearly, the radical interpretive approach, as outlined above, breaks new grounds in research on conspiracy theories. Its iconoclastic allure is partly down to the fact that under this model, the analysis does not have to be limited to the acts of the ascription of conspiratorial thinking (which are performed in the casual, political, or media contexts), but may be further extended to cover similar practices under the psychological approach, which reproduces the principles of commonsense reasoning in this respect.

20 Similar anti-cognitivist theories are advocated by representatives of so-called discursive psychology, but from the perspective of ethnomethodological conversation analysis, discursive psychology does not fully deliver on its anti-psychological promise in research practice (Button, Lynch & Sharrock, 2022, 133–138).

However, adopting the radical interpretive approach to analysing conspiracy theories is not without problems, because in this approach, evaluative judgements are avoided, while exclusive focus is given to the reconstruction of the rules of ascribing conspiratorial thinking to others. One obvious question arising at this point is whether phenomena such as conspiracy theories may be exempt from similar judgments, and arguments for answering this question in the negative appear very compelling: to use a popular example, abstaining from judgment on this count would lead to the unjustified blurring of the distinctions between charging captain Dreyfuss with allegedly conspiring against the state and Emile Zola's open letter accusing members of the French top military brass of the actual conspiracy against Dreyfuss. In other words, it would be hardly acceptable to systematically ignore the communicative, political, and moral differences between inaccurate and accurate conspiracy theories, even if proving their formal similarities could be cognitively valuable. To be sure, bandying around the term of "conspiratorial thinking" is potentially harmful. Still, impartiality favoured under a third approach does little to reduce the risks involved.

6. Conclusions

In May 2023, the World Health Organization announced that the COVID-19 pandemic was over. However, this announcement did not put an end to the conspiracy theories concerning the sources of the pandemic, its course, and the large-scale vaccination campaign launched to soften its impact. On the contrary, the COVID-related conspiracy theories, especially those which openly promote the view (or at least insinuate) that COVID vaccination is harmful, have been on the rise and proliferated on the Internet. In early 2024, a familiar sequence of events unfolded: an international team of researchers published the results of studies conducted across a record-large sample of 99 million study subjects, which revealed that adverse events following vaccination were very rare (Faksova et al., 2024). It was not long before the Internet spawned stories questioning these findings in the spirit of tailor-made conspiracy theories. Given their immense popularity, any attempts (such as those by David Gorski, 2024) to debunk them by refuting their supporting pseudo-arguments are unfortunately doomed to fail.

None of this means that professional virological research is unnecessary – actually, it is absolutely critical. It is as critical to make science-based efforts toward dispelling conspiracy theories. At the same time, it is time to accept that even highly credible studies and extremely compelling criticism of conspiracy theories will not only fail to win over their proponents, but also see them become even more entrenched in their positions. Conspiracy theories enjoy success not because of a lack of proper research or scholarly counterarguments, but due to the paradoxes and pitfalls involved in social communication.

One important aspect of this situation appears to be the contrast between the immense persuasive force of conspiracy theories and an insufficient meta-reflection upon the state of their scholarly analyses. I have tried to demonstrate that a scholarly analysis of conspiracy theories should join forces with a scholarly – i. e. distanced and self-critical – meta-reflection, and the latter may lead to re-formulating the method of studying conspiratorial thinking. The present article is an attempt toward that end, and this is precisely why both approaches have been interlaced throughout.

Appropriate in summation would be a pointing out of the theoretical and practical conclusions drawn from the remarks presented herein. Inferences of a theoretical nature should begin from a constatation that schematism is a ubiquitous tendency in the academic process. With reference to sociology, Loïc Wacquant spoke of radical forms of schematism in the form of epistemic "bandwagons" and "turnkey problematics":

> [S]ocial scientists are always in danger of falling for a turnkey problematic, that is, a set of prepackaged categories, questions, methodological moves and data banks encapsulated by a term, often promulgated by research agencies, public bureaucracies, political officials, and private philanthropies to suit their own agendas, or propelled by the mere routine of professorial reproduction. A turnkey differs from the disciplined application of paradigmatic principles in that it invites the routinized and unthinking implementation of a rhetorical and technical formula whose social parameters are taken for granted by scholars and officials alike. (Wacquant, 2022, 87)

There is no reason for the same dangers not to exist in psychology and social psychology. Furthermore, or so it seems, a psychological approach to studies into conspiracy theories does meet the definition of a "turnkey problematic" about which Wacquant spoke.

Fusing the features of conspiracy theories and of the theories of conspiracy theories, the objective in this text has been to show two primary research approaches – not only the traditional, still dominant psychological analysis of conspiracy theories, but also an analysis of conspiratorial culture that focuses on social mechanisms. Pointed out, too, have been new possibilities that the analysis of the communicative aspects of conspiracy theories has opened up for the field of research on conspiracy culture. Logically, as these gain a stronger foothold in the field of conspiracy studies, descent into a "turnkey problematic" begins to jeopardise the cultural approach. Yet the horizon of such a state of affairs is still far off in the distance. Until that becomes a closer reality, the cultural approach provides new, novel, albeit controversial impulses in the field of conspiracy theory analysis.

Formulated in several places in this text are concrete, practical recommendations regarding advisable and inadvisable ways of talking about pandemic issues. As it turns out, these ways of talking about such matters fall into three relatively distinct categories. The first layer is simply about how to talk and not talk about the coronavirus contagion and its consequences. Nevertheless, the list of practical issues does not end here. As I have also tried to show, reflections on how to speak of the virus, and the pandemic it sparked, inevitably lead to the question of how to talk about COVID-19-related conspiracy theories. In other words, what are the arguments in favour of talking about conspiracy theories in psychological, cultural, and/or interpretive terms? Finally, a separate, third layer relates to how to talk and not talk to backers of conspiracy theories about the pandemic. Generally speaking, it can be said that the divides outlined herein can serve to organise discussions not only with respect to the COVID-19 plague, but also other social problems. The following scheme could serve us well:

- How to speak (or not) about a social problem (i.e., how to speak or not about the COVID-19 pandemic)?;
- How to speak (or not) about clichéd communication patterns regarding a social problem (i.e., how to speak or not about conspiracy theories on the subject of the coronavirus pandemic)?; and
- How to speak (or not) with supporters of a rote pattern of communication about a social problem (i.e., how to speak or not with advocates of conspiracy theories on the subject of the COVID-19 pandemic)?

Partial answers to these questions are scattered across the present article. However, they do not coalesce into a comprehensive and uniform set of guidelines, and in addition, inadvisable ways of talking about pandemic issues receive more attention than advisable ways of talking about it. This is hardly surprising, seeing as conspiracy theories tick all the boxes of a "wicked problem": they are such a complex and multifaceted issue that no clear consensus exists over how to define it or what measures to take against it. Furthermore, attempts at solving the problem of conspiracy theories (or any other "wicked problem") usually lead to unanticipated consequences, while the issue of conspiracy theories itself is relentless, in that "it cannot be solved 'once and for all'" (cf. Weber & Khademian, 2008). Thus, analysing conspiracy theories and finding ways of counteracting them require a self-critical approach and receptiveness to new ideas.

The suggested shift of analytical focus toward the communicative aspects of conspiracy theories is consistent with a similar change (proposed elsewhere) in understanding political culture. Under the traditional model, political culture is defined through the prism of citizens' and politicians' respective motivations, attitudes, or personality traits, and studying it falls within the purview of political psychology. On the other hand, in a communicational approach, political culture concerns patterns of public communication about public issues, and as such becomes a subject of rhetorical criticism and discourse analysis (cf. Czyżewski, 2014). Obviously, conspiracy theories are also in private circulation and – together with hate speech and other negative tendencies – contribute to the erosion of communication culture in general. The significance of the quality of public communication about public issues belongs to a different dimension of collective life: said quality determines the standard of political culture, and the latter is a litmus test of modern democracy.

Works cited

Anton, A. & Schink, A. (2021). *Der Kampf um die Wahrheit. Verschwörungstheorien zwischen Fake, Fiktion und Fakten.* München: Komplett Media GmbH.

Aupers, S. (2012). "Trust No One". Modernization, Paranoia and Conspiracy Culture. *European Journal of Communication* 27/1, 22–34. doi: 10.1177/0267323111433566.

Bachmann-Medick, D. (2016). *Cultural Turns. New Orientations in the Study of Culture.* Boston: De Gruyter.

de Balzac, H. (2004). *The Lost Illusions.* London.

Barkun, M. (2003). *A Culture of Conspiracy. Apocalyptic Visions in Contemporary America.* Berkeley: University of California Press.

Barkun, M. (2013). *A Culture of Conspiracy. Apocalyptic Visions in Contemporary America*, 2nd Edition. Berkeley: University of California Press.

Bauman, Z. (2017). *Wasted Lives. Modernity and its Outcasts.* Cambridge: John Wiley & Sons.

Billig, M. (1991). *Ideology and Opinions. Studies in Rhetorical Psychology.* London: SAGE Publications.

Bodner, J., Welch, W., Brodie, I., Muldoon, A., Leech, D. & Marshall, A. (2021). *Covid-19 Conspiracy Theories. QAnon, 5G, the New World Order and Other Viral Ideas.* Jefferson, NC: McFarland.

Bogner, A. (2021). *Die Epistemisierung des Politischen. Wie die Macht des Wissens die Demokratie gefährdet.* Ditzingen: Reclam.

Boltanski. L. (2014). *Mysteries and Conspiracies: Detective Stories, Spy Novels and the Making of Modern Societies.* Cambridge: Polity.

Bormann, E. G. (1984). *The Force of Fantasy: Restoring the American Dream.* Carbondale Il: Southern Illinois University Press.

Bourdieu, P. (1991). *Language and Symbolic Power.* Cambridge: Polity Press.

Bourdieu, P. & Wacquant, L. J. D. (1992). *An Invitation to Reflexive Sociology.* Chicago: The University of Chicago Press.

Bratich, J.Z. (2008). *Conspiracy Panics. Political Rationality and Popular Culture.* New York: State University of New York Press.

Butter, M. (2020). *The Nature of Conspiracy Theories.* Cambridge: Polity Press.

Butter, M. (2022). *Teorie spiskowe. Nic nie jest takie, na jakie wygląda.* Kraków: Wydawnictwo Uniwersytetu Jagiellońskiego.

Butter, M. & Knight P. (2019). The History of Conspiracy Theory Research: A Review and Commentary. In J.E. Uscinski (ed.), *Conspiracy Theories and the People Who Believe Them* (pp. 33–46). Oxford: Oxford University Press.

Butter, M. & Knight, P. (eds.) (2020). *Routledge Handbook of Conspiracy Theories.* London: Routledge.

Button, G., Lynch, M. & Sharrock, W. (2022). *Ethnomethodology, Conversation Analysis and Constructive Analysis. On Formal Structures of Practical Action.* London: Routledge.

Carver, B., Craciun, D. & Hristov, T. (eds.) (2020). *Plots. Literary Form and Conspiracy Culture.* London: Routledge.

Czech, F. (2015). *Spiskowe narracje i metanarracje.* Kraków: Nomos.

Czyżewski, M. (1989). Garfinkel, "Cognitive Revolution" and Conversation Analysis. *International Journal of Sociology of Language*, 78, 43–55. doi.org/10.1515/ijsl.1989.78.43.

Czyżewski, M. (2014). Praca pośrednicząca w debatach publicznych. In M. Czyżewski, K. Franczak, M. Nowicka & J. Stachowiak (eds.), *Dyskurs elit symbolicznych. Próba diagnozy.* (pp. 380–409). Warszawa: Wydawnictwo Akademickie SEDNO.

Czyżewski, M. (2018). A Brief Outline of Issues Related to the Democratisation of Culture: A Contemporary Perspective. *Societas/Communitas*, 2–3, 43–60.

Czyżewski, M. (2023). Single Case as an Object of Analysis. In Defense of a Species Threatened with Extinction. In Ł. Kumięga & M. Nowicka-Franczak (eds.), *Analysing Discourse, Analysing Poland. The Case of a Political Interview* (pp. 25–55). Göttingen: Vandenhoeck & Ruprecht Verlag.

Dentith, M.R.X. (ed.) (2018). *Taking Conspiracy Theories Seriously.* London.

Douglas, K.M. (2021). COVID-19 Conspiracy Theories. *Group Processes & Intergroup Relations*, 24, 2, 270–275. doi.org/10.1177/1368430220982068.

Eglin, P. (1978). What Should Sociology Explain – Regularities, Rules or Interpretations? *Philosophy of the Social Sciences*, 5, 377–391. doi:10.1177/004839317500500302.

Fairclough, N. (2013). *Language and Power*, 2nd edition. London: Routledge.

Faksova, K. et al. (2024). COVID-19 Vaccines and Adverse Events of Special Interest: A Multinational Global Vaccine Data Network (GVDN) Cohort Study of 99 Million Vaccinated Individuals. *Vaccine*, 12, 02. doi.org/10.1016/j.vaccine.2024.01.100. https://www.sciencedirect.com/science/article/pii/S0264410X24001270.

Ferguson, N. (2017). *The Square and Tower: Networks, Hierarchies and the Struggle for Global Power.* London: Penguin.

Fleck, L. (1981). *Genesis and Development of a Scientific Fact.* Chicago: University of Chicago Press.

Foss, S.K. (2018). *Rhetorical Criticism: Exploration and Practice*, 5th edition. Long Grove, Il.: Waveland Press.

Foucault, M. (2003). *Society Must Be Defended. Lectures at the Collège de France, 1975–1976.* New York: Picador.

Garfinkel, H. (1963). A Conception of, and Experiments with, "Trust" as a Condition of Stable Concerted Actions. In O.J. Harvey (ed.), *Motivation and Social Interaction* (pp. 187–238). New York: Ronald Press.

Garfinkel, H. (1967). *Studies in Ethnomethodology.* Englewood Cliffs: Prentice-Hall.

Gorski, D. (2024). How Antivaxxers Weaponize Vaccine Safety Studies to Falsely Portray Vaccines as Dangerous. *Science-Based Medicine* 26.02. https://sciencebasedmedicine.o

rg/how-antivaxxers-weaponize-vaccine-safety-studies-to-falsely-portray-vaccines-as-dangerous/ (26 March 2024).

Graumann, C.F. & Moscovici, S. (eds.) (1987). *Changing Conceptions of Conspiracy*. New York: Springer-Verlag.

Harambam, J. (2020). *Contemporary Conspiracy Culture. Truth and Knowledge in an Era of Epistemic Instability*. London: Routledge.

Hristov, T. (2019). *Impossible Knowledge. Conspiracy Theories, Power, and Truth*. London: Routledge.

Hofstadter, R. (1966). The Paranoid Style in American Politics. In idem, *The Paranoid Style in American Politics and Other Essays* (pp. 3–40). New York: Alfred A. Knopf.

Jaskułowski, P. (2019). *The Everyday Politics of Migration Crisis in Poland: Between Nationalism, Fear and Empathy*. Cham: Palgrave Macmillan.

Lord, Ch.G. , Ross, L. & Lepper, M.R. (1979). Biased Assimilation and Attitude Polarization: The Effects of Prior Theories on Subsequently Considered Evidence. *Journal of Personality and Social Psychology*, 37, 11, 2098–2109.

Madisson, M.L. & Ventsel, A. (2021). *Strategic Conspiracy Narratives. A Semiotic Approach*. London: Routledge.

Mannheim, K. (1956). The Democratization of Culture. In idem, *Essays on the Sociology of Culture* (pp. 171–246). London: Routledge.

Melley, T. (2002). Agency Panic and the Culture of Conspiracy. In P. Knight (ed.), *Conspiracy Nation. The Politics of Paranoia in Postwar America* (pp. 57–81). New York: NYU Press.

Mierzyńska, A. (2021). Milionowe zasięgi, pikniki, koncerty i petycje. Polscy przeciwnicy szczepień to rosnący problem. *OKO.press*. Retrieved 19 July 2021, from https://oko.press/polscy-przeciwnicy-szczepien-to-rosnacy-problem.

Otrocki, M. (2017). *Dyskurs spiskologiczny. O racjonalność w metajęzyku krytycznym*. Wrocław: Wydawnictwo – Drukarnia PHUP "eRKa – PRINT" Roman Kolasa.

Pacewicz, K. (2021). Tylko jedna czwarta Polek i Polaków odporna na argumenty antyszczepionkówców [Sondaż]. *OKO.press*. https://oko.press/tylko-jedna-czwarta-polek-i-polakow-odporna-na-argumenty-antyszczepIonkowcow-sondaz-oko-press (16 May 2021).

Pacewicz, P. & Piechowicz, Z. (2016). Katastrofa smoleńska. 24 teorie spiskowe. *OKO.press*. https://oko.press/katastrofa-smolenska-24-teorie-spiskowe (06 July 2016).

Pickel, G., Öztürk, C., Schneider, V. , Pickel, S. & Decker, O. (2022). Covid-19-Related Conspiracy Myths, Beliefs, and Democracy-Endangering Consequences. *Politics and Governance*, 10,4, 177–191. doi:10.17645/pag.v10i4.5798.

Pilch I., Turska-Kawa, A., Wardawy, P., Olszanecka-Marmola, A. & Smołkowska-Jędo, W. (2023). Contemporary Trends in Psychological Research on Conspiracy Beliefs. A Systematic Review. *Frontiers in Psychology*, 14, 1–19. doi: 10.3389/fpsyg.2023.1075779.

Shils, E.A. (1996). *The Torment of Secrecy: The Background and Consequences of American Security Policies*. Chicago: Ivan R. Dee.

Stachowiak, J. (2023). Użytkowe własności wypowiedzi prawdziwościowej. Myślenie spiskowe i prawda w dyskursie publicznym. *Przegląd Socjologiczny*, 4, 57–82. doi: 10.26485/PS/2023/72.4/3.

Uscinski, J.E. & Parent, J.M. (2014). *American Conspiracy Theories*. Oxford: Oxford University Press.

Wacquant, L. (2022). Epistemic Bandwagons, Speculation, and Turnkeys. *Thesis Eleven*, 173, 1, 82–92. doi:10.1177/07255136221121705.
Watson R. & Coulter, J. (2008). The Debate over Cognitivism. *Theory, Culture &Society*, 25, 2, 1–17. doi: 10.1177/0263276407086788.
Weber, E.P. & Khademian, A.M. (2008). Wicked Problems, Knowledge Challenges, and Collaborative Capacity Builders in Network Settings. *Public Administration Review*, 68, 2, 334–349. doi.org/10.1111/j.1540-6210.2007.00866.x.
Weisbrod, L. (2022). Müssen wir anders mit Verschwörungstheorien umgehen? *Zeit Online.* https://www.zeit.de/kultur/2022-07/verschwoerungsanhaenger-umgang-impfgegner-querdenker?utm_referrer=https%3A%2F%2Fwww.google.com%2F (10 July 2022).
Wetherell, M. & Potter, J. (1992). *Mapping the Language of Racism: Discourse and the Legitimation of Discrimination.* New York, NY: Columbia University Press.
Zamorski, M.A., Komenda, K. & Przekora, K. (2021). *Wielki reset. Jaką przyszłość planuje nam globalna władza. Dokumenty z komentarzem.* Wrocław: Wydawnictwo Wektory.
Zamorski, M.A. (2020). *Operacja pandemia. Globalna psychoza i nowy totalitaryzm.* Wrocław: Wydawnictwo Wektory.

Thomas Niehr

What Linguistics Has to Say about Conspiracy Theories[1]

Abstract
This article examines what specific contribution linguistics can make to the assessment of conspiracy theories. Linguistic methods of argumentation analysis are of particular interest here. After an introductory clarification of terminological issues, Stephen Toulmin's argumentation model, which is widely used in linguistics, is introduced and proves helpful in assessing existing argumentations. Finally, examples are given to show that conspiracy theorists often use argumentative methods which, on closer inspection, are not very convincing and cast considerable doubt on the rationality of the argumentation in question. The ability to analyse arguments with regard to their rationality thus proves to be indispensable in order not only to classify conspiracy theories as such but also to see through them.

Keywords: conspiracy theory, argumentation analysis, contradiction, collective knowledge, coronavirus pandemic.

1. Introduction

Conspiracy theories have boomed during the coronavirus pandemic. This is clear to anyone who, even fleetingly, has noticed reports about "lateral thinking" demonstrations, or has been confronted with corresponding theories on social media. It is not at all clear to what extent the number of conspiracy theories has increased recently. The uncomplicated "viral" dissemination methods available via digital communication channels may be responsible for the impression that conspiracy theories are circulating everywhere. These seem to be focusing on the

Thomas Niehr, RWTH Aachen University, ORCID: 0000-0001-6704-9464.

1 The following is a translation of an article originally published in German and has not been changed or updated: Niehr, T. (2022), Was die Linguistik zu Verschwörungstheorien zu sagen hat. In Eleftheriadi-Zacharaki, Sofia et al. (eds.), *Vom Umgang mit Fake News, Lüge und Verschwörung. Interdisziplinäre Perspektiven.* Baden-Baden: Nomos, 105–120.

coronavirus pandemic at the moment. In fact, there have been and continue to be other thematic areas where conspiracy theories are circulating.

The following article will explore the question of the specific contribution which linguistics can make to the assessment of conspiracy theories. However, it must first be clarified to what extent linguistics is at all suited to judging conspiracy theories – or more precisely: to judging whether a theory is rightly labelled a conspiracy theory.

2. Why linguistics?

If you wish to answer the question of to what extent it might be natural to draw on findings from linguistics when it comes to assessing whether something is a conspiracy theory or is rightly labelled as such, then one argument is obvious: theories – of whatever kind – must be verbalised in order to be disseminated in a society or in parts of society. Such verbalisations can be oral or written, or even oral and written. However, as soon as verbalisation has taken place, there is a (verbal and/or written) text, be it large or small. And one of the genuine tasks of linguistics is undoubtedly to analyse the nature of texts.[2]

In our context, the structure of such texts, which are labelled as conspiracy theories, is of particular interest. One could ask, for example, whether such texts are characterised by a common structure and how this structure can be described. First of all, however, a terminological question needs to be clarified. The term *conspiracy theory*, which is also widely used in colloquial language, appears problematic when it is used to characterise texts in linguistic or even scientific terms. This is because it is a pejorative term that would appear unsuitable for the factual description of a text. Contemporary linguistics sees itself, to a large extent, as a descriptive science that describes language but does not evaluate it.[3] If terms such as *conspiracy theory*, *empty phrase*, *buzzword* or *euphemism*, which are often used in a derogatory way in colloquial language, are to be suitable for the linguistic categorisation of linguistic phenomena, a precise definition is required that makes it possible to distinguish them from colloquial connotations.[4] Such a

2 Text linguistics is a sub-discipline of linguistics. It deals with "the production, structure, function and processing of texts" (Glück & Rödel, 2016, s.v.). Brinker, Cölfen & Pappert (2018) provide a good introductory overview.

3 One exception to this is linguistic language criticism, which – partly based on rhetorical principles – makes criticism-led statements about the appropriateness of language use; see Kilian, Niehr & Schiewe (2016) and Niehr, Kilian & Schiewe (2020).

4 For the definition and use of the terms *buzzword* and *empty phrase* in linguistics, see Niehr (2007, 2019a). On *euphemism*, see Niehr (2019b). For criticism of the term *conspiracy theory*, see also Römer & Stumpf (2020, 252–253).

definition can be successful if it is based on linguistic categories, because linguistics is not limited to describing and analysing grammatical regularities, but also takes into account the characteristics of text types, modes of argumentation and linguistic strategies. A typical question for linguistics in this context, which will be pursued in the following section, could therefore be aimed at the extent to which conspiracy theories are characterised by linguistic similarities.

3. Linguistic characteristics of conspiracy theories

When we talk about conspiracy theories later, we will do so with the proviso that we are dealing with a colloquial expression whose meaning initially remains somewhat vague. Thus, unpopular points of view, in which, for example, a possibly justified mistrust is given expression, are often discredited as conspiracy theories, which are based on harmful conspiracy thinking. In this way, the term *conspiracy theory* becomes a term of delegitimisation that can be used almost at will to counter opposing arguments. In colloquial [German] language, this is also known as a "Totschlagargument", i.e. an argument that does not address the matter under discussion but is generally designed to end the argument in favour of the person dubbing it a conspiracy theory.

A further difficulty with the term is related to the second (right-hand) part of the compound term *conspiracy theory*. The term *theory* has a precise meaning, especially in scientific contexts. The same applies to terms such as *method* or *hypothesis*. However, if we look at typical uses of the term *conspiracy theory*, it becomes very clear that the components of *theory*[5] that are meant in scientific contexts obviously cannot be intended.

However, Römer and Stumpf (2020, 252) rightly point out that *theory* is also used colloquially in another sense, namely as a "notion alien to reality; mere conjecture" (Duden, 2019, 1786)[6].

It can therefore be seen that the colloquial meanings of the term *conspiracy theory* make it difficult to determine its precise meaning.

Despite these difficulties, an attempt can be made to describe the linguistic commonalities of conspiracy narratives. In the following, we will draw on two different approaches that address different characteristics of conspiracy narratives. In his approach, Michael Butter (2018) focuses in particular on the specific argumentation of conspiracy theories:

5 For example, the Duden Universal Dictionary defines theories as "a system of scientifically based statements to explain certain facts or phenomena and the laws underlying them" (Duden 2019, 1786).

6 All of the German-language quotations in this article have been translated into English by the editors of the volume.

Conspiracy theories claim that a group operating in secret, namely the conspirators, is trying to control or destroy an institution, a country or even the whole world for base motives. (Butter, 2018, 21)

The base motives mentioned in this quote are of particular interest in our context. This term, which is used in the German Criminal Code (Section 211) to evaluate motives for murder and is often criticised not only because of its Nazi origins but also because it cannot be operationalised, means that acts are "no longer humanly comprehensible or understandable, even in the broadest sense" (Bosch, 2015, 804). This brings categories such as "unrestrained libidinous selfishness" or "blatant selfishness" (cf. ibid.: 804–805) into play. Such motives are also attributed to the alleged conspirators. Added to this is the motive of self-interest:

> Conspiracy theorists always tell history from the end. They ask who benefits from an event or a development and thus identify those who must be responsible for it. They believe in a mechanistic view of the world in which there is no room for chance, unintended consequences or systemic effects. For them, observable events are the effects of intentional actions and make it possible to infer the motives of the actors. (Butter, 2018, 59)

To draw such conclusions, argumentative procedures are required, which, according to a common definition, are used to "transform something collectively questionable into something collectively valid" (Klein, 1980, 19). The peculiarity of conspiracy theory argumentation, however, is that this process is usually reversed: Something that is (almost) collectively valid is to be called into question or even proven to be collectively invalid (cf. section 5.3 below).

This can easily be illustrated with a current example. During the coronavirus pandemic, it should be widely recognised that we are dealing with an extremely dangerous viral infection for which there is currently no effective medication. It therefore seems sensible to vaccinate as many people as possible against the virus in order to prevent further infections and contagions or to mitigate the consequences of an infection.

If we look at conspiracy narratives surrounding the coronavirus pandemic against this background of collective knowledge, it becomes clear that this is precisely where they start. In line with the approach described by Butter, the story is told "from the end" and the question is posed as to who could be benefitting from the pandemic and the measures taken to combat it. This question is answered in different ways but the answers always lead to similar results: An elite is always identified as benefiting from the pandemic – be it the pharmaceutical industry, Bill Gates making money from vaccinations, or various "politicians" who want to permanently restrict our basic rights, abolish cash or introduce compulsory vaccination.

However, the existence of such similarities says nothing about the correctness or plausibility of the underlying argumentation. Using a model known in argumentation theory, the following section therefore attempts to uncover typical, i. e. exemplary, argumentation weaknesses in conspiracy narratives.

4. Argumentation and its structure

The British philosopher of language Stephen Toulmin published the book "The Uses of Argument" in 1958. Toulmin's theory of argumentation, in particular his model of argumentation, has been popular in Germany since the 1970s and has since become a classic.[7] There are several reasons for this. The most important is probably that Toulmin very clearly recognises the uselessness of formal logic when it comes to evaluating real argumentation. This is because formal logic emphasises the form of an argument without taking its content into account. In particular, syllogisms whose conclusion is already contained in the premises[8] have little to do with everyday argumentation, in which we are dependent on conclusions of a completely different kind:

> We make claims about the future, and back them by reference to our experience of how things have gone in the past; we make assertions about a man's feelings, or about his legal status, and back them by references to his utterances and gestures, or to his place of birth and to the statutes about nationality; we adopt moral positions, and pass aesthetic judgements […]. Whenever we do any of these things, there can be no question of the conclusion's being regarded as a mere restatement in other words of something already stated implicitly in the datum and the backing […]. (Toulmin, 2003, 115–116)

Against this background, Toulmin presents the components of an argument as follows:

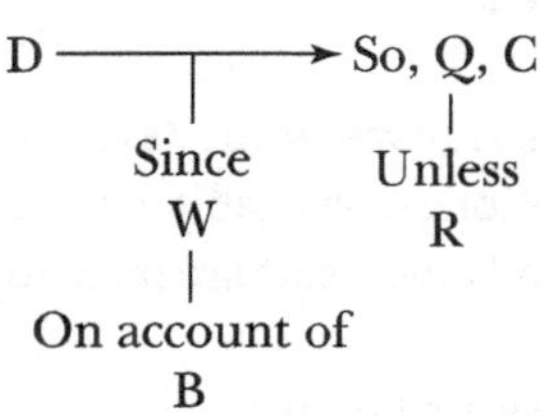

Fig. 1: Abstract Toulmin scheme (Toulmin 2003, 97).

7 Toulmin's model has also been criticised and further developed. For reasons of space, these will not be pursued further here; cf. the handbook articles with references by Kienpointner (2017) and Niehr (2017) on this and on more recent forms of argumentation analysis.

8 In particular, a syllogism of the type "All men are mortal. Socrates is a human being. Therefore Socrates is mortal", in which the conclusion follows directly from the premises.

Starting from a conclusion (C), we can ask which datum (D) this conclusion is based on. The transition from the datum to the conclusion is made possible by a warrant (W), which may need to be justified by a backing (B). Optionally, a rebuttal (R) and a modal qualifier (Q) can be added. If this scheme is filled with statements, the result is, for example:

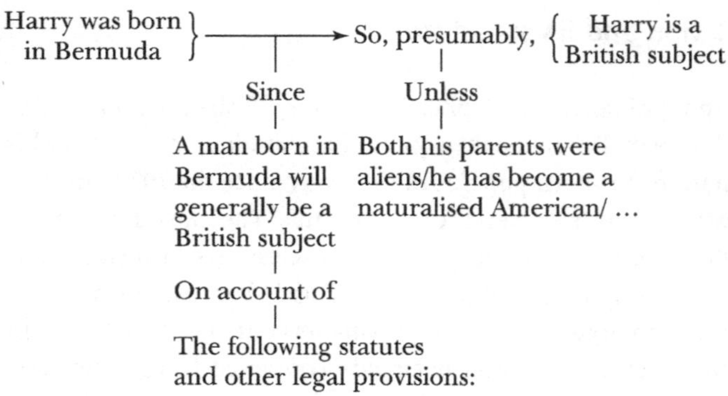

Fig. 2: Concrete Toulmin scheme (Toulmin, 2003, 97).

The quality of an everyday argument can be assessed with relative certainty based on such a schema. Although not all positions in the schema have to be filled (cf. Niehr, 2017, 170), they should at least be reconstructable without great effort for reasonable, well-meaning recipients. This applies in particular to the rule of inference, which usually remains implicit and guarantees the transition from the data to the conclusion and thus the plausibility of a concluding procedure not only in formal terms.

5. The argumentation of a conspiracy theorist

Drawn from the rich pool of circulating conspiracy narratives, some texts by Heiko Schrang are used below. Some of them are no longer available on the Internet because Schrang frequently changes websites and older texts are then no longer available.

Among other things, Schrang runs a homepage (www.heikoschrang.de) and his own YouTube channel, called SchrangTV.[9] He has been agitating there for some time against "politicians" whom he accuses of conspiring against the people. This conspiracy is also evident in various measures taken to tackle the coronavirus pandemic, which he claims are actually being taken to curtail peo-

9 On Schran's other activities, see Niehr (2021). SchrangTV can be found at: https://www.youtube.com/user/SchrangTV.

ple's rights, abolish cash and gain total control over the population with the help of RFID chips that are implanted during coronavirus vaccinations. Before the pandemic, Schrang came out with claims that were also directed against political measures in a conspiracy theory manner. For example, he claimed that reunification had only been undertaken to abolish the Deutschmark.

In our context, the main area of interest is the argumentative support for such claims. Various argumentative patterns can be identified here, each of which is illustrated by an example below.

5.1 *Post hoc ergo propter hoc*

The concept described in the title of this section is considered a fallacy in rhetoric. It consists of deducing causality (Latin: *propter hoc*) from a temporal sequence (Latin: *post hoc*) or correlation. This figure corresponds with the assertion on which conspiracy theories are often based that there are no coincidences, that everything is somehow connected to everything else. Conspiracy theorists often claim to see (hidden) connections that remain hidden from average people. Heiko Schrang uses this technique several times in his reflections on the Bilderberg conferences[10].

> The fact is that in recent decades, especially after the Bilderberg events, noticeable changes have taken place (the introduction of the euro, the Lehman Brothers bankruptcy, the Ukraine crisis, the refugee crisis and many more). To the uninformed, 'coincidental' events with enormous significance for the world economy and global development have repeatedly occurred following Bilderberg conferences in recent years. In mid-2008, for example, the conference met in Washington and a few months later the investment bank 'Lehman Brothers' was allowed to fall by the wayside. The following year, a meeting was held in Athens and a short time later the Greek debt crisis began, the after-effects of which we are still feeling today. In any case, it is astonishing that enormous career leaps have repeatedly taken place after Bilderberg events. One such example is Christian Lindner, whose FDP is being widely celebrated after elections in North Rhine-Westphalia and is supposed to offer AfD voters a 'more democratic' alternative for Germany. What few people realise, however, is that Christian Lindner became the new leader of the FDP in 2013 after making his debut at the Bilderberg meeting just a few months earlier.[11]

If we analyse this line of argument using the Toulmin scheme, the following structure emerges:

Datum: Changes of global significance occurred after Bilderberg conferences.

10 On the conspiracy theory potential of the Bilderberg conferences, see Niehr (2020, 156).

11 Heiko Schrang: EILMELDUNG: Soll Trump weg? Bilderberger-Treffen 2017 in den USA, http://www.macht-steuert-wissen.de (22 May 2017).

Conclusion: Changes, some of them of global significance, were planned and decided at Bilderberg conferences and then implemented.

It is no coincidence that it is difficult to formulate a plausible warrant that could ensure the transition from the datum to the conclusion. One possible formulation could be as follows:

Warrant:

If changes of sometimes global significance occur after Bilderberg conferences, then they were planned, decided and implemented there.

The following could then be used to back the warrant:

If two events/developments A and B occur in immediate temporal succession (and/or local proximity), it is not a matter of coincidence, but rather A is the cause of B or B is the effect/consequence of A.

It seems obvious that neither the formulated warrant nor the backing can claim general validity. Otherwise, it would be possible to construct any number of correlations, provided there was a temporal sequence (and/or local proximity), irrespective of the contextual relationships. Examples include weather changes (as a result of political influence), pandemic outbreaks (as a result of technical developments such as 5G or Wi-Fi technology) or negative stock market developments (as a result of weather changes). Although such connections cannot be completely ruled out by means of rational argumentation, the formulated warrant is obviously not suitable for enabling a rationally justified transition from the given datum to the conclusion. Instead, it is used to justify assertions that Butter (2018, 22), following the American political scientist Michael Barkun, characterises as basic assumptions of conspiracy theory arguments:

> "1) Nothing happens by chance.
> 2) Nothing is as it seems.
> 3) Everything is connected."

These basic assumptions can be read as a set of guidelines for uncovering conspiracies. Initially, this requires adopting a fundamentally sceptical stance that continually seeks out hidden powers operating behind the scenes–powers capable of making events or developments, orchestrated for their own benefit, appear to the broader public as mere coincidences. If this is indeed the case, it becomes only natural to strive to look beyond the pervasive facade and see through the evoked appearance. Should one succeed in doing so, numerous hidden interconnections emerge that must be exposed in order to neutralise the conspirators' schemes.

5.2 The argumentum from authority

This argumentation style is characterised by the fact that an authority/authorities are used to support the argument in question. In order to assess such an argument, it is crucial to determine which authority is used for which thematic area and whether the authority selected can actually claim authority status in the relevant subject area. A look at arbitrarily constructed examples shows that the plausibility of an authority argument is not always a given.

If, for example, a humanities scholar is cited as an authority on medical issues, she is not very convincing as an authority, even if she has academic titles. The same applies if a person who is controversial in specialist circles and who is known to hold outsider opinions is to act as a witness for far-reaching claims in this specialist field. However, such weaknesses are typical of the authority arguments put forward in conspiracy theories.

For example, conspiracy theorists repeatedly cite doctors as authorities on virological issues. In particular, the pneumologist and former head of the Flensburg Health Department dr Wolfgang Wodarg[12] and the emeritus professor of medical microbiology dr Sucharit Bhakdi[13] should be mentioned here. Both have put forward theses relating to the coronavirus pandemic that can be characterised as (scientifically) outsider opinions. This alone, however, should cast doubt on their authoritative status in questions of virology.[14]

Claims that can be heard time and again from such experts involve assertions that coronaviruses have been known for a long time and are no more dangerous than influenza viruses, at the moment there is a lot of scaremongering going on, and that vaccination is pointless at best, but dangerous at worst.[15]

Looking at the key thesis of this argument using the Toulmin scheme reveals the weakness of this conclusion, regardless of whether medical experts are cited to confirm it:

Datum: Coronaviruses are not new, but have been known for a long time.
Conclusion: Coronaviruses are not dangerous.
Warrant: Known viruses are not dangerous.

12 Further information on Wodarg's career can be found in the corresponding Wikipedia article: https://de.wi-kipedia.org/wiki/Wolfgang_Wodarg (15 April 2021).

13 More information on Bhakdi in the corresponding Wikipedia article: https://de.wikipedia.org/wiki/Sucha-rit_Bhakdi (15 April 2021).

14 The Duden universal dictionary defines an authority as a "personality with significant influence and a considerable [professional] reputation" (Duden 2019, 250).

15 Cf. for example the correction by Correctiv: https://correctiv.org/faktencheck/hinter-grund/2020/03/18/coronavirus-warum-die-aussagen-von-wolfgang-wodarg-wenig-mit-wissenschaft-zu-tun-haben/ and https://correctiv.org/faktencheck/2020/06/19/impfung-gegen-covid-19-sinnlos-sucharit-bhakdi-stellt-unbelegte-behauptungen-auf/ (22 April 2021).

If you start with the warrant when assessing this conclusion, it proves to be implausible. A reference to smallpox, HIV or polio viruses may suffice at this point to illustrate their non-validity (and dangerousness). With the unacceptability of the warrant, however, the entire argument loses plausibility. The weakness of such an argument cannot be compensated for by the fact that alleged authorities agree with it.

5.3 The argument of contradiction

Conspiracy theories often aim to transform something collectively valid into something collectively questionable, as has already been stated above. In order to achieve this, they must be counter-arguments that are directed against claims to validity that are largely undisputed. An effective argumentative means of delegitimising opposing validity claims is to prove contradictions in the argumentation of the opponent. If this succeeds, the plausibility of the opponent's argument is shaken, and with it often the credibility of the opponent.

However, the decisive factor in this line of argument is what exactly is to be regarded as contradictory. This is where a diachronic component comes into play, which is often paraphrased in everyday German language with the saying "What do I care about yesterday's gossip" ["Was stört mich mein Geschwätz von gestern?"]. This saying criticises the inconsistency of statements made by a person at different times. However, the time difference is of crucial importance here. This is because absolutizing the demand for consistency between a person's statements would turn any change of opinion and even any progress in learning into a contradiction and thus, indirectly, into a credibility problem. In particular, if the demand for freedom from contradiction does not relate to individuals but to collectives, such as "politics" or "science", it can be used strategically.

Heiko Schrang, for example, takes advantage of this in his video of 21 April 2021[16]. There, he criticises a contradiction in the fact that pupils are now obliged to take rapid Covid tests before attending school. Until that point ("still at the beginning of last year"), however, it had been claimed that children were not severely affected by this virus and would not pass it on.[17]

---

16 It is entitled "Willkommen in der Diktatur!". The quoted passage begins in the 9th minute of the video, which can be found at the time of writing at https://www.heikoschrang.de/de/neuigkei-ten/2021/04/19/21-april-willkommen-in-der-totalen-diktatur/ (23 April 2021).

17 Similar "contradictions" can be seen in experts' recommendations as to which coronavirus vaccines should preferably be used for which groups of people. They are a clear example of how gaining knowledge can lead to uncertainty. In this particular case, this uncertainty seems to have led many people to judge the potential risks of vaccination with the active ingredient

In this passage, Schrang deliberately ignores the fact that science (in this case, virology) also continues to develop and can arrive at new findings that make new measures appear sensible or even necessary. If this fundamental fact is ignored, it is easy to uncover alleged contradictions. However, such contradictions, which are often blamed on "politics", can only undermine the credibility of the opponent as plausible arguments "if the systematic claim to the consistency of such statements is able to relativise the time difference of their utterance as an irrelevant contextual determination" (Kopperschmidt, 1989, 198–199). However, this does not apply to scientific statements in particular, since the essence of science is to put theories and hypotheses up for discussion and, ideally, to arrive at new insights by testing and, if necessary, refuting them.

Germany's Health Minister Jens Spahn summed up this fact in a debate in the Bundestag on 22 April 2020, by stating the following:

> I completely agree with you on something else – and I also want to say this in principle about other debates, for example on masks and other things – namely that we will probably have to forgive each other a lot in a few months, because never before –
> (Laughter from members of the Left Party)
> – Yes, you may laugh, but I will say it anyway – in the history of the Federal Republic of Germany and perhaps beyond, such far-reaching decisions have never had to be made in such a short space of time under such circumstances with the knowledge that is available and with all the uncertainties that exist. I am always envious of those who have always known everything.
> We have all learnt a lot together in recent weeks, including about this virus and some of the consequences of decisions. I am sure that beyond politics, there will also come a time for society, even for virologists and scientists, where we will all realise in retrospect that we may have been wrong in one place or another or that we will have to correct and readjust things in one place or another. I think that's relatively normal at a time like this. If we had a fundamental understanding that this is part and parcel of a time of such unpredictability, then that would be an important step.
> (German Bundestag – 19th electoral term – 155th session. Stenographic report, p. 19211, B)

On closer inspection, the demand for freedom from contradiction thus proves to be an argument that can by no means claim blanket validity. Particularly in the case of collectives whose diversity is often disguised with generic terms such as "politics" or "science", freedom from contradiction cannot be demanded as a sign of transparency or credibility in the naïve understanding outlined here.

---

from Astra Zeneca to be higher than the dangers of infection with the coronavirus. (At least this was the case at the time this article was finalised early in May 2021).

6. Conclusion

This article has used selected examples to illustrate that conspiracy theories are linguistic constructs that utilise special argumentative procedures. Such procedures play a central role in conspiracy theories because conspiracy theories are essentially counter-arguments that are directed against the validity claims of collectively valid constructions of reality.

By analysing the arguments, it can be shown that the plausibility of conspiracy theory arguments is doubtful. The lack of plausibility is due to erroneous conclusions or persuasive procedures that do not fulfil the criteria of rational argumentation or even deliberately undermine them. It therefore requires the competence to scrutinise argumentation for its rationality to see through conspiracy theories for what they actually are – argumentative sleight of hand, which, when viewed in the cold light of day, by no means emanate the "peculiarly unconstrained compulsion of the better argument" (Habermas, 1971, 137).

Works cited

Bosch, N. (2015). Niedrige Beweggründe. *JURA – Juristische Ausbildung*, 37, 8, 803–812. DOI: 10.1515/jura-2015-0162.

Brinker, K., Cölfen, H. &Pappert, S. (eds.) (2018). *Linguistische Textanalyse. Eine Einführung in Grundbegriffe und Methoden.* 9, durchgesehene Auflage, Berlin: Schmidt (= Grundlagen der Germanistik, Bd. 29).

Butter, M. (2018). *Nichts ist, wie es scheint. Über Verschwörungstheorien.* Berlin: Suhrkamp (Edition Suhrkamp Sonderdruck).

Duden (2019). *Deutsches Universalwörterbuch. 9., vollständig überarbeitete und erweiterte Auflage.* Berlin: Dudenverlag.

Glück, H. & Rödel, M. (eds.) (2016). *Metzler Lexikon Sprache.* 5., aktualisierte und überarbeitete Auflage. Stuttgart: Metzler.

Habermas, J. (1971). Vorbereitende Bemerkungen zu einer Theorie der kommunikativen Kompetenz. In N. Luhmann & J. Habermas (eds.), *Theorie der Gesellschaft oder Sozialtechnologie* (pp. 101–141). Frankfurt am Main: Suhrkamp.

Kienpointner, M. (2017). Topoi. In K.S. Roth, M. Wengeler & A. Ziem (eds.), *Handbuch Sprache in Politik und Gesellschaft* (pp. 187–211). Berlin/Boston: de Gruyter (Handbücher Sprachwissen, 19).

Kilian, J., Niehr, T. & Schiewe, J. (2016). *Sprachkritik. Ansätze und Methoden der kritischen Sprachbetrachtung.* 2., überarbeitete und erweiterte Auflage. Berlin/Boston: de Gruyter (Germanistische Arbeitshefte, 43).

Klein, W. (1980). Argumentation und Argument. In *Zeitschrift für Literaturwissenschaft und Linguistik* (38–39), pp. 9–57.

Niehr, T. (2007). Schlagwort. In G. Ueding (ed.), *Historisches Wörterbuch der Rhetorik.* Band 8: Rhet – St. (pp. 496–502), Tübingen: Niemeyer, S. Niehr, T. (2017). Argumentation in Texten. In Sven Roth, K., M. Wengeler & A. Ziem (eds.), *Handbuch Sprache in Politik und Gesellschaft*, (pp. 165–186). Berlin/Boston: de Gruyter (Handbücher Sprachwissen, 19).

Niehr, T. (2019a). Schlagwörter und Leerformeln in der politischen Rede. In A. Burkhardt (ed.), *Handbuch Politische Rhetorik* (pp. 671–688). Berlin/Boston: de Gruyter (Handbücher Rhetorik, 10).

Niehr, T. (2019b). Euphemismus – (k)eine Kategorie der linguistisch-deskriptiven Diskursanalyse? In Rocco, Goranka/Schafroth, Elmar (eds.), *Vergleichende Diskurslinguistik. Methoden und For-schungspraxis. In Zusammenarbeit mit Juliane Niedner* (pp. 93–112). Berlin: Peter Lang (Kontrastive Linguistik / Linguistica contrastiva, 9).

Niehr, T. (2020). Populistische Medienkritik im Netz. Erscheinungsweisen und Erklärungsversuche. In K. Beckers & M. Wassermann (eds.), *Wissenskommunikation im Web. Sprachwissenschaftliche Perspektiven und Analysen* (pp. 141–161). Berlin [u. a.]: Peter Lang (Transferwissenschaften, 11).

Niehr, T. (2021). Argumentation und Narration in verschwörungstheoretischen Youtube-Videos. In *Zeitschrift für Literaturwissenschaft und Linguistik*. DOI: 10.1007/s41244-021-00203-5.

Niehr, T., Kilian J. & Schiewe, J. (eds.) (2020). *Handbuch Sprachkritik*. Stuttgart: Metzler.

Nocun, K. & Lamberty, P. (2020). *Fake Facts. Wie Verschwörungstheorien unser Denken bestimmen*. Köln: Quadriga.

Römer, D. & Stumpf, S. (2020). Sprachliche Mittel in Verschwörungstheorien. Das Beispiel "Gates kapert Deutschland". In *Der Sprachdienst* 64, 6, pp. 249–259.

Toulmin, S. (2003): *The Uses of Argument*. Cambridge, U.K/New York: Cambridge University Press.

Discourse and Epistemic (B)orders

Giampietro Gobo

The Decline of Trust towards Scientists after COVID-19. A Pilot Study in the Italian Context[1]

Abstract
The COVID-19 pandemic has once again highlighted the long-standing issue of trust in science and scientists. Many approaches, however, tend to either analyse science as a fully autonomous entity – attributing the decline in trust to external factors – or treat trust as a binary concept, considering it either present or absent. Instead of assuming a straightforward causal relationship from external influences to science itself, this article adopts perspectives that explore how science interacts with other social subsystems.
The goal is to offer a more nuanced approach that moves beyond binary distinctions, such as those between internal scientific processes and external societal factors – distinctions often implied in terms like "infodemic," "disinformation," or "pseudoscience." To achieve this, two research directions were pursued. First, the study examined two expert conflicts that shaped public debate in Italy during the SARS-CoV-2 outbreak, requiring scientists to engage with different social subsystem logics. Second, a pilot study was conducted on a sample of online readers from two Italian newspapers to move beyond a binary understanding of trust and explore attitudes toward science and scientists.
The findings reveal a more complex perspective on trust in scientists, identifying five distinct attitudes influenced by both how scientists communicate and the underlying philosophy of science they convey in media interactions.

Keywords: COVID-19, trust in science, secularisation of science, expertise, attitudes towards science, scientism.

1. Introduction

A massive exposure in the media of virologists, biologists and scientists mostly dealing with health occurred in Italy from February 2020 due to the COVID-19 pandemic. This occurrence made them more known and popular; however, it

Giampietro Gobo, University of Milan, ORCID: 0000-0002-3519-5640.
1 The preparation of this paper was supported by the Department of Philosophy "Piero Martinetti" of the University of Milan within the project "Departments of Excellence 2018–2022," awarded by the Ministry of Education, University and Research (MIUR).

may also have signalled the beginning of an unexpected decline in public trust towards them and their fields of study, as shown by a pilot study (survey) conducted in 2021.

Hence, a scientistic and positivist vision of science has begun to crack, as testified by the fact that a consistent element of people (between 20% and 30%, so still largely a minority) seems to share a constructivist epistemological model, unmoored to presumed certainties and absolute truths (typical of scientism), and more focused on conflicts between knowledge and a continuous questioning of acquired knowledge.

This phenomenon, based on the responses of the interviewees, does not seem to be, at least in the first instance, the product of a delegitimisation of science coming from the world of social media, but rather the result of the media exposure of scientists: precisely, as scientism (largely present in the mainstream media) has made excessive promises, the disillusionment in discovering that they have not always been kept may have contributed to generating a sceptical attitude of part of the population (a minority, but growing).

In addition, it would seem that just the traditional media, with their mediatisation of the conflicts between scientists and experts, have contributed to the strengthening of this critical sentiment towards scientists, which we could define as the "secularisation of science".

2. Scientistic culture and its possible downsizing

Scientism generally defines an intellectual attitude whereby scientific knowledge must be the foundation of all knowledge, even in ethics and politics. From February 2020, during the COVID-19 pandemic, citizens were asked to largely rely on science on more than one occasion, thus foreshadowing a sort of technocratic government. A perspective that seems to refer to the solution of any problem (scientific, social, political, ethical) to the "experts," supposedly the only ones with the right knowledge to face any situation and resolve it. One of the many indicators of the scientist attitude is the wide use in public discourse of expressions such as "unscientific," "natural," "objective," "factual," "true truth," "pseudoscience," "conspiracy theories," "fake news," and "post-truth" (Habgood, 2019): a group of terms aimed at providing a reassuring vision of science, conceived of as a business with precise boundaries and unequivocal results (Gobo & Marcheselli, 2022). However, this stereotypical portrait does not reconcile itself with the intrinsic presence of inevitable controversies, divergent theses and plural perspectives.

Friedrich von Hayek, a sociologist and 1974 Nobel Laureate in Economics, was among the first to criticize scientism: in his *Scientism and the Study of Society* (divided into three parts, published in 1942, 1943 and 1944, respectively) he disputed the application of natural science methods to the study and solution of problems relating to social institutions and the community. Later, Karl Popper, referring to Hayek himself, foresaw the presupposition of totalitarianism in the methodological dogmatism that was typical of scientism. According to Popper, science proceeds not only rationally but also with the help of other forms of thought such as, for example, metaphysics. Furthermore, the philosopher was also sceptical about the fact that any certainty could be reached in the scientific field without renouncing the search for truth, this being the presupposition of his critical rationalism. Finally, Popper pointed out the inconsistency of concepts such as the much-invoked "scientific method," as the presumed objective criterion for evaluating a theory: "there is no scientific method in any of these three senses: [...] there is no method to discover a scientific truth; there is no method to assess the truth of a scientific hypothesis, that is, no method of verification; there is no method to assess whether a hypothesis is *probably true*" (Popper, 2009, 44). Philosophers such as Hilary Putnam (1992) and Cvetan Todorov (2001), and the sociologists Max Horkheimer and Jürgen Habermas have long fought scientism, considered as a cultural phenomenon to be the child of modern Western civilization. But perhaps the staunchest opponent of scientism was Paul K. Feyerabend. Although at a young age he started out from scientistic positions, later he became convinced that science is "an essentially anarchist enterprise" and did not deserve any exclusive monopoly on the "business of knowledge."[2]

This demand for certainty partly expressed by scientism is also inherent in the peculiar relationship of mutual dependence between specialists and the public. In this regard, Ludwik Fleck (1986) had already analysed this relationship in terms of a dynamic between an esoteric circle (which the specialists belong to) and an exoteric one, composed of a wider audience accessing the knowledge produced by the first circle only through the mediation of the specialists themselves. The latter tend to be assertive and to simplify their positions in their interacting with the laymen, and in their attempt to make themselves understood. Those belonging to the exoteric circle, in turn, tend to take as dogmas the statements of the specialists they trust, and ask them for further certainties. Thus, according to Fleck, due to this peculiar dynamic (and, according to us, given the high levels of trust towards specialists) when an idea passes from the esoteric to the exoteric circle, it necessarily becomes less complex and acquires a degree of certainty greater than the one it had within the esoteric circle of competence. Conse-

2 It should be noted, however, that the scientistic attitude is often present also in the scholars and researchers accused of being charlatans, impostors and pseudoscientists. In fact, they in turn consider their opponents to be ignorant, incapable or, worse, in the pay of industry and multinational corporations. In other words, both factions often take scientistic and neo-positivist positions.

quently, both the spread of the infection and the media exposure of scientists further fuelled a social demand for certainty, which science has long been subjected to, a demand destined to remain unfulfilled, particularly in the early stages of the virus' circulation.

Furthermore, despite the fact that the so-called "information deficit model" – that paternalistically reduces the problem of greater or lesser confidence in science to a question of its being poorly understood by the public – has long since been largely viewed as outmoded in specialist literature (Bucchi & Neresini, 2008), it remains the tacit reference model in the practice of scientific communication.

Thus, the scientific debates on TV have in a sense "unveiled" a series of dynamics that, heretofore familiar only to the fields of philosophy and the sociology of science, concerned the temporary and conflictual nature of scientific acquisitions. If, on the one hand, science revealed itself to the general public with a new face, i. e. as an entirely "human" and "social" enterprise, on the other hand, a gap was generated between science "as it is" and "how it should be". In fact, while showing itself to be litigious and conflictual in media debates, science was invested by the same media with a demand for epistemological and social certainty that it could not satisfy.

All these elements may have contributed to a downsizing of the scientistic attitude (still dominant today), and to the emergence of a different epistemological model among the general public, a new image of science, of the Kuhnian and partly also Popperian type (to the detriment of the neo-positivist model): comprised of conflicts, interests, different opinions, certainties that are called into question after a few weeks, predictions that do not always come true, correct and incorrect therapies, etc. This is an epistemological model that (according to our hypothesis) could undermine the scientistic model among the general public.

Therefore, there are various signs of a *downsizing* of scientism, i. e. a greater caution in accepting uncritically what scientists say. This, as we have seen, should not be ascribed to a wrong way of proceeding on the part of scientific knowledge during the pandemic, but to the gap generated between what "science should be" (the request for monolithic certainties, also promoted by the mainstream media) and what it actually "is" (its inherent provisional nature, which manifested itself during the pandemic, particularly in the first phase), together with the intensification of conflicts due to the choices made by the media themselves.

It is precisely this disillusionment with respect to an ideal model of science, strongly linked to the mediatisation of the scientific debate, that could therefore explain a partial (we repeat, only partial, but that in the future could be destined to worsen) decline in trust toward scientists.

3. The decline of trust in scientists

According to a survey carried out at the end of October 2020 by *Observa – Science in Society* (https://www.observa.it/), between the first pandemic wave (March 2020) and the second one (October 2020), the positive judgment towards scientific experts dropped by 23 percentage points, "thus squandering the large consensus accumulated in the spring." In fact, one in four Italians gave them a negative rating. One reason can be found, according to the responses in the survey, in the "media overexposure of national scientific experts increasingly perceived as a source of confusion, was lamented in October by 62% of citizens compared to 48% in March; [moreover] fewer than a fifth of Italian citizens consider the communication of experts to be clear and effective, and a tenth would prefer they advise political decision-makers confidentially, and not publicly" (Bucchi, 2021).

Before the spread of Sars-Cov-2, as attested by the International Science Survey 2019–2020 conducted by the Pew Research Center in Washington, the level of trust towards scientists in Italy was relatively high: 76% of respondents declared they had a lot of trust (33%) or a fair amount of trust (43%), while 20% said they had little or no trust in scientists. Data from 3M's State of Science Index created by the Ipsos Institute between February and March 2021, and thus two months before our survey, are more complex to interpret. Despite very high levels of agreement with the direct statement "I trust science" (91% of respondents were completely or fairly in agreement with the statement, whereas 10% were in disagreement),[3] there were other elements that seem to go in the opposite direction. For example, 16% answered to be sceptical of science and 24% to be unsure whether scientific research was conducted according to ethical principles.

Thus, generally speaking trust in scientists is still high; nevertheless, the phenomenon of its decline is worrying being mistrust likely to increase rather than decrease in the future. In fact, once lost, trust – always been somewhat of a scarce resource – is difficult to recover.

3 It is surprising that the percentage of "I don't know" responses or unanswered questions is not given, though always present in a survey and sometimes showing a very high percentage. On what basis the percentages were calculated is therefore not known. Note that a fair number of non-responses would cause the sample to lose representativeness; in fact, depending on the number of non-responses and how they are treated statistically, the percentages could change, even significantly. If they were included in the count, the percentages based on the answers would decrease. On the other hand, if they were excluded, relying only on the so-called "valid percentage" would produce a fictitious increase in the opinions expressed, especially in favour of those in the majority. Thus the (actual) results of the Italian Ipsos research may perhaps not differ so much from those of our research.

A pilot study

In order to further reveal attitudes towards science and scientists, we conducted a pilot study[4] on a sample[5] of online readers of *Il Fatto Quotidiano* and *The Post Internazionale* (TPI)[6]. The following reflections are therefore only valid for the readers of these two newspapers and cannot be generalized to the Italian population, even if they seem consistent with the results of other national sample surveys reported above. Thus, from 10 to 17 May 2021, 3,391 and 587 questionnaires were collected, respectively, for a total of almost 4,000 standardised online interviews.

The questionnaire of the web-survey (which cannot be fully included here for limited reasons of space) was intended to detect attitudes towards scientists, doctors in particular, and the image of science held by respondents. Some of its total 13 questions, whose average completion time was 12 minutes, were original, while others were taken from surveys previously conducted by other survey institutes in order to attempt a comparison. Among the original questions, some were formulated from statements expressed on TV by well-known scientists or journalists. Others (especially those relating to science) were drawn from statements by important philosophers of science (such as Popper, Hanson and

4 A pilot study can be defined as an initial application, on a small scale, of a study protocol, in order to check whether the project is adequate, establish its feasibility, or obtain information that permits the remedy of inconsistencies and errors, so as to design a subsequent study with a representative sample.

5 This study is not based on a representative sample of the Italian population. The differences with a sample of that type are many. First of all, interviewees were readers of online newspapers (in Italy there are still many people who do not read a newspaper); then, most of them are politically oriented towards the left, the centre-left and the Five Star Movement; and have a much higher education than the average member of the Italian population. Finally, the presence of the male gender is overrepresented. In particular, males were 67% and females 31%, while 2% did not respond. Furthermore, 11% of the sample was between 14 and 34 years old, 31% between 35 and 54 years old, 27% between 55 and 64 years old, and 31% over 64 years old. With regard to educational qualifications, 41% of the sample had a diploma or high school diploma, 19% a degree in scientific subjects, and another 18% a degree in the humanities; 12% had a doctorate or other specialization. 32% of readers lived in the north-west, 22% in the north-east, 24% in the centre, 13% in the south, 8% in the islands and 1% abroad.

6 Recruitment took place through the publication of an article on the home page of *Il Fatto* and *TPI*. The same article was then also published on the Facebook pages of the two newspapers. Here is the text of the article (written in order to make the request as neutral as possible): "Scientists and the pandemic. The SARS-COV- 2 pandemic made the widespread communication of scientific information about COVID by the mass media necessary. We saw many scientists on TV shows and read many of their interviews in newspapers and online newspapers. We would like to understand your thoughts about this new phenomenon: did the presence of scientists in the media help you to better understand the various issues concerning the virus? What is your opinion of science and scientists? Your answers will be useful for university research on the perception of science during the pandemic."

especially Feyerabend). Finally, we included many control questions to test the coherence and stability of respondents' opinions.

To gather information on the SARS-CoV-2 virus and the COVID-19 disease, TV programmes were the primary source used by respondents (48%); followed by newspapers, both in print and online, (19%); the Internet – Google, Wikipedia, YouTube – (11%); institutional websites – of Regions, of the Ministry of Health, etc. – (4%); general practitioners (1%); blogs and forums (0.6%); family members and friends – also via chat – (0.4%). Surprisingly, 9% of respondents stated they did not use any source (among the many listed in the question), and only 3% of them declared the much discussed social media (Facebook, Twitter, WhatsApp, Telegram, Signal, Instagram, etc.) to be their main source. Certainly, the latter data point is partially due to the fact that online-newspaper readers were interviewed. However, the contiguity of the mode used (online), which also includes social media, might have led to imagine a higher percentage.

What do interviewees think: a methodological problem as well

An interesting (and methodologically relevant) aspect that emerges from the survey is that a share of respondents (around 20–25%) seems to be keen to distinguish between science and scientists, i. e. between science "as it is" (the behaviour of scientists) and how it "should be" (the ideal of science). From a sociological point of view this would seem to be a poor distinction, as scientists are those that make science: science as an abstract entity does not exist. Yet this distinction can, at least partially, explain apparently contradictory results. A similar phenomenon can in fact be found in a survey published on 21 February 2021, carried out by the company Sigma Consulting, on a representative sample of 700 residents of the Italian region Marche. While, on the one hand, respondents declared themselves to have great faith in science, on the other, two thirds of them relied or had relied upon alternative and/or complementary medicines that most scientists and doctors often declare to be ineffective.[7] Therefore, there seems to be a cognitive dissonance in a significant proportion of respondents: on the one hand there is a "good" science that is both objective and impersonal, and on the other hand there are "bad" scientists that apply it badly. But can science exist independently from scientists?

Faced with this phenomenon, it is possible to react in at least two ways. One way could follow what Henri Laborit, a French biologist, loved to argue, i. e. the

7 The data point could also be interpreted by suggesting that respondents believe that alternative and/or complementary medicines are fully part of science. From this perspective, what sounds like a contradiction to the researcher no longer is.

beliefs guiding the life of human beings are a messy jumble of clichés and stereotypes, without coherence, and of little value. Indeed, Converse (1964 and 1970) held that only a minority of people (less than 4%) exhibited stable and consistent attitudes, while the majority have a reduced and fragmented belief system (1964, 247). The former possess well-structured attitudes, while the latter have non-attitudes (Converse, 1970).

However, Sudman, Bradburn and Schwarz later criticised the "non-attitude" concept on the grounds that "human reasoning is always context-dependent" (1996, 125), it is indicative, as Garfinkel would say (Garfinkel, 1967). According to Krosnick and Abelson, the five dimensions that characterise stable attitudes are: extremism, emotional intensity, security, subjective importance, and knowledge (1992). Consequently, few people are quite so *rigid.* On the other hand, most do not always have well-defined values and preferences and it often happens that though we prefer Y, yet we reject it because opinions and social values are subordinated to the specific request of the test or questionnaire (Shafir, Simonson & Tversky, 1993).

With this in mind, it is notable that a portion of the sample (ranging between 30% and 37%) has a critical and generally negative judgment of how scientists behaved during the spread of the virus' spread. It is a minority percentage, though it deserves attention. More worrying, however, was the fact that only 43% of respondents agreed on the substantial consistency of the scientists' statements, while 56% found them to be often contradictory.

Scientism, realism, constructivism, disenchantment and anarchism: five images of science

It makes no sense to continue providing percentages as the sample under survey is not representative of the whole Italian population. Thus, it is more interesting to try and piece together the structure of reasoning that guides attitudes towards science and scientists. Five main attitudes emerged through an exploratory factor analysis[8], which explain 51.6% of the variance[9].

8 Factor analysis (both exploratory and confirmatory) is a set of statistical techniques used to search for the existence of latent dimensions (or factors), starting from a series of observed variables. They are said to be latent because, despite being the organizing fulcrum of the variables, they are not directly detectable. The objective of this analysis is to understand whether these detectable variables are effectively and consistently attributable to that underlying dimension (concept) which by its nature cannot be directly detected.

9 Variance is a measure of dispersion or variability of a data set or frequency distribution. It is used to know how far the different scores of a variable are from the mean of the same (and therefore if the mean is a good synthetic indicator for that phenomenon we are trying to detect). The higher the value, the greater the variability; the lower the value, the more ho-

A first latent dimension is the one linked to a certain *scepticism, disillusionment* and *disenchantment*. This is based on the belief that "many scientists said things that are imprecise and of which they had only partial competence" (61%); they made "overly peremptory statements, without even adding a 'maybe' or 'it could be'" (62%); they (those appearing on TV) appeared to be "fortune tellers rather than scientists" (35%). The fact that "many scientists have become TV stars, spending more time on the screen than in the lab or hospital following patients" (61%) also seemed to disturb people. Furthermore, it was assumed that "scientists do not always tell the truth, because they constantly depend on industry money" (46%). As such, "because of their knowledge, scientists have a great power that makes them dangerous" (24%), and so, "although science was born as a liberation movement, today it has become an oppressive ideology" (22%), thereby retracing the thinking of Feyerabend.

A second dimension, which contrasts with the first, was represented by those who shared a *scientistic and positivist attitude.* This dimension belonged to the majority of respondents and was based on the certainty that "science is science, and has no political colour" (81%) as well as on the statement that "scientists act rationally and on the basis of data and evidence" (86%). There was a belief that "most scientists proved themselves to be competent" (65%) and "their interventions made me more informed and my knowledge increased" (64%). Therefore, "it is important that more and more scientists go on TV" (59%). This attitude holds that "scientific knowledge must be the foundation of all knowledge in any sphere of society, even in ethics and politics" (77%) and thus "politicians must follow the opinion of scientists and experts" (84%). Finally, "a doctor who decides NOT to be vaccinated against the SARS-Cov 2 virus should change their job" (87%).

A third attitude is what we might define as *realist* which, despite having contiguity with the previous one, is distinguished (even philosophically – Popper for example) from a scientistic vision. It believes in objectivity ("the truths of science are NOT contaminated by the beliefs of the moment, because they are objective and impersonal" – 67%), but has an elitist conception of science as "scientific knowledge cannot be communicated to ordinary people, because their contents are too complex" (17%) and "any problem (scientific, social, political, ethical, etc.) must be dealt with by experts, because they are the only ones who have the suitable knowledge to deal with and solve it" (63%).

mogeneous the measurement will be. The more an underlying dimension (see note 4) is able to reduce the variance, the more we have compactness, coherence and homogeneity in the data set. So, by "explained variance" we mean that portion (hopefully as large as possible) which is clarified, resolved, illuminated by the underlying dimension identified.

A fourth dimension is the *constructivist* attitude, in which science is seen as an enterprise that traces, in all respects, the strengths and weaknesses of human action. As for its merits, "science does not proceed only rationally, but also through other ways of thinking (e. g. imagination, intuition, creativity, etc.)" (65%). With regard to its defects, "even natural sciences (e. g. physics and chemistry), and not only human sciences (e. g. sociology and anthropology), are also influenced by the personal beliefs and opinions of scientists" (29%) and thus share the position of American feminist philosopher Sandra Harding (1986), who argued that physics, chemistry, mathematics and logic bear the cultural imprints of their creators, no less than anthropology and history. As a consequence, even "experiments are always influenced by the historical period in which they are carried out (given by the prejudices of the scientists, the techniques and technologies they used and the beliefs of the time, etc.)" (65%). However, it is not just (albeit important) cultural influence. There is also intentionality, because "much of the scientific knowledge we have today is the result of partisan interests" (42%) and "scientists, when they express their evaluations, are sensitive to what politics has to say" (33%). Finally, "scientific knowledge can be communicated to ordinary people, but scientists often do not know how to communicate it" (74%).

The last relevant dimension, more than the previous one, embodies an *anarchic and tolerant vision* of science, proposed by Feyerabend in the seventies and according to which "in science it is necessary to give a voice to everyone, even to points of view that at that moment may seem wrong" (73%). Consequently, "all beliefs, even those of a religious nature, can participate in the scientific debate" (21%). Furthermore, "it is advisable to conserve all theories, even those that have been discarded over time, because it is always possible they will become current again" (58%). Finally, "a doctor who does NOT visit at home a patient who may suffer from Covid, should change their job" (77%).

In general, however, it can be affirmed that the absolute majority of respondents (between 50 and 60%) possess a convinced scientistic and positivist view of science, in which they do not see a distinction between science and scientists. A minority (between 15 and 20%), on the other hand, that shares an idealistic and romantic image, regrets the gap between science and scientists, and when asked to take sides in a semantic differential often places itself halfway, among the uncertain (as per table 1); finally, another minority (between 20% and 30%) has a historicised, critical and cultural vision of science.

Education: are the critics and sceptics ignorant?

Another *topos* is that critics and sceptics of science are the least educated people. This is the thesis, among many others, of Achterberg and colleagues (2017). Differently, in our study, whose interviewees were online-newspaper readers implying a certain education, scientistic thinking appears to be more prevalent among less educated people. According to our data, previous research on members of critical movements about childhood vaccinations (Lello, 2020) and biotechnologies (Bucchi & Neresini, 2002), which state that those members have rather high levels of education and information. Probably, data and questions crafted in the questionnaires are influenced by biases of the researchers themselves, who tend to consider science as a uniqueness rather than a plurality of knowledge and methods.

Political orientation: is critical thinking towards science right-wing?

It has often been repeated that critical thinking towards science (erroneously called "anti-scientific") lurks in the right, especially the extreme one. For example, according to a research conducted before the 2020 epidemic by the aforementioned Pew Research Center in Italy, trust in scientists is often greater in people with a centre-left political orientation (47% of these respondents have "a lot of trust" in scientists against 31% of those on the centre-right).

Our pilot study, however, offers some data that allows us to question some established interpretations. In fact, only 6% of our sample declared to be centre-right, while the rest stated to be from the extreme left (7%); left (38%); centre-left (23%), and centre (6%); then, 11% did not recognise themselves in any of these labels, and 8% considered themselves non-partisan or apolitical.

This leads us to three considerations:

- that the critical component towards scientists, which is relevant even in a sample composed primarily of people politically oriented towards the left or centre-left, is underestimated in the national research conducted on representative samples;
- that, if we could have reached a greater number of center-right respondents, the number of critics would probably have increased;
- that questions about trust in scientists are often too simplistic, strongly indicative, and fail to adequately discriminate the thoughts of respondents.

Hence, an added value of this pilot study is to investigate the scepticism also present on the left, guiltily neglected by the representations of most of the media.

Scientists versus Constructivists

The conceptual differences between proponents of scientism and constructivists were also expressed by different positions regarding the scientific method, the democratic nature of science, conflicts of interest and the boundaries of science (see Table 1). It should be noted that in the face of a clear predominance of scientistic positions, constructivist ones also make up a significant percentage and should not be underestimated.

Table 1: Combined percentages of the 7-position semantic differential.

	Adherents of scientism	**uncertain**	constructivists	
There is only one science, based on a SINGLE method, based on experiments	56%	10%	34%	There is NOT ONLY ONE science, but MANY different sciences, based on different methods
Science is NOT democratic, because it is the facts that impose themselves on the attention of scientists; beyond what most of them might think	46%	15%	39%	Science is democratic because it is the majority of scientists who decide among the many existing facts, which to study and which to verify
The boundary between science and non-science is clear and precise	54%	13%	33%	The boundary between science and non-science is uncertain and continuously redefined
Most scientists work for the common good	44%	15%	41%	Most scientists have conflicts of interest

The secularisation of science

In their reflections, some important sociologists such as Weber, Troeltsch, and Durkheim have given wide space to the phenomenon of secularisation. Durkheim, for example, believed that modernity would lead traditional religion into irreversible decline; however, he was also convinced that every society needed that connective texture (made up of values, beliefs, ceremonials and rituals capable of enacting strong feelings and bonds of solidarity) provided by religion. Therefore, in highly differentiated societies, such as contemporary ones, religion would not have disappeared, but would have undergone a transformation, consisting in the secularisation of its contents (the sacralisation of the human person and the cult of the individual, as Goffman would later admirably show). Secularisation, therefore, means the phenomenon whereby a society (or part of it) moves away from traditional cultural models, as well as from dogmatic and *a priori* positions based on authority. To this end, it is worth mentioning that, in informal conversations in the late 1980s, the philosopher and anthropologist of science Bruno Latour used to provocatively repeat that fewer and fewer people believed in God and practiced a religion, and that the only religion left was science. Now, according to the research presented above, we are perhaps witnessing a renewed phenomenon of the secularisation of science. Renewed because it had already appeared in the 1970s and continued until the first decade of the 2000s, when critical thinking was more developed (think of the followers of the Frankfurt School, postmodern criticism and the Alterglobal movement of radical opposition to scientistic neoliberalism). In more recent years, we have witnessed a return of scientism that reached its peak in the first months of the spread of the virus. We could therefore say that there are two opposing tendencies that coexist and alternate in our societies: that of scientism (majority) and the one of the secularisation of science (now minority). They are unfortunately creating phenomena of polarisation of opinions (see Gobo & Sena, 2022).

A clue: adherence to the anti-Covid 19 vaccination campaign

An indicator of the decline of trust in scientists can be found in the initial low adherence of people to the vaccination campaign, actually started in Italy on 1 January 2021. As of 31 March, only 9,928,663 had been vaccinated, i.e. 20% of the population over 20 and many had already booked their first shot of the vaccine. However, the next day, with the executive order of 1st April, the first vaccination obligation was imposed on doctors, nurses and all healthcare personnel. It seems strange that it was necessary to resort to obligation precisely for professionals who are in greater contact with medical-scientific knowledge. As of 15 April, there were about 13,900,000 (23%) vaccinated and as of 30 April, about 19,400,000 (33%). A second obligation, the so-called "Green Pass", was introduced in Italy on 1 July 2021. Beyond the dubious health effectiveness of this tool as a barrier to contagion (in fact, in the winter of 2022 infections reached peaks of 200,000 infected per day, despite the fact that most of the Italian population was vaccinated), it immediately seemed to push people to get vaccinated, as publicly declared by some Italian ministers. Only on that date and with other obligations arriving (in September for teachers and then gradually for other categories), 87% of the population over 20 were vaccinated. The slow progress of vaccinations and the introduction of Green Pass obligations highlight that (along with calls for responsibility, altruism, the common good, and the fear of getting sick) one of the main factors that led to the success of the vaccination campaign was precisely the reinforcement of the Green Certificate. Hence, the decision to get vaccinated does not seem to mainly depend on people's trust in science, rather on their need not to lose some fundamental civil rights such as freedom to access shops; rights of movement, residence and expatriation; of meeting, working and receiving a salary. Thus, these kinds of policies may have had the effect of increasing distrust of science.

A further confirmation of this analysis lies in the trend, following the termination of the obligation, of people's compliance with the fourth dose of the vaccine. Although strongly recommended by the majority of scientists, advised by the government and sponsored by the mainstream media, "the administration of the fourth doses (second booster) has undergone a rapid decline for months, shows very low coverage rates particularly in the Southern Regions and leaves uncovered 11,9 million people", as noted by the Gimbe Foundation (press release, 6 February 2023).

4. Conclusion: Where were scepticism and a crisis of expertise born?

Summarising this pilot study, we can state that the absolute majority of the interviewees (ranging between 50% and 60%) possess a convinced scientistic and positivist vision of science, in which they see no distinction between science and scientists. A minority (ranging between 15% and 20%), sharing an idealistic and romantic image, regrets the hiatus between science and scientists, and, when asked to take sides in a semantic differential, often places themselves somewhere between the uncertain (see table 1). Finally, another minority (ranging between 20% and 30%) has a historicised, critical and cultural vision of the science. Let us focus on the latter group.

The great media exposure, probably unprecedented, has made public a question hitherto relegated only to science studies: who are the experts? (Collins & Evans, 2002; Shapin, 1988; Epstein, 1995; Jasanoff, 2005) These studies had already highlighted how expertise, i. e. professional competence, is not simply a resource attributed to a single individual (however "special" it may be), but to a group, of which the individual is recognised as a member. Over time, the problem of competence has become more and more problematic, as witnessed by the titles of the most recent books: Collins and Evans (2007) *Rethinking Expertise*; Eyal (2019) *The Crisis of Expertise*; Nichols (2017), even more *tranchant*, *The Death of Expertise.* The topic of competence has therefore re-emerged in the face of multiple conflicts (not only of interpretation) among scientists. However, the research results raise doubts about recent theories that assign a strong role to social networks and fake news in the ever-increasing diffusion of so-called anti-scientism (Moran, 2020). Surely (and our survey also reveals it) the most critical people of science and scientists are frequent users of social networks. However, very few people use them as a primary source (3%). Hence, our hypothesis that it is precisely the traditional media (primarily TV), in which there is a widespread scientism also reinforced by the request for certainty addressed to scientists by television presenters, that feed (indirectly and unknowingly) a growing critical attitude towards science, which can also border on anti-scientific sentiment. Widespread scientism and critical/anti-scientific attitude, in part, are both the consequence of forecasts (statistical and otherwise) that have not come true (Campo et al. 2021); of the disorientation and confusion in the public opinion following the television conflicts between scientists; of the disillusionment in discovering that some promises of emergency exit have not been maintained. Notably, some of the long-standing unresolved problems of medicine are in the list given (see Lello, 2020; Hornsey, Lobera & Díaz-Catalán, 2020).

Moreover, the dynamics of conflict have to be taken into account; although inherent in the scientific debate, they have been amplified by the spectacularisation processes of science that took place during the pandemic. Although the public visibility of some scientists is not a new phenomenon, the pandemic has given the scientific community unprecedented media exposure. Furthermore, the same media have largely "rewarded" the scientists who are best known and most visible in the public debate, as well as tending to behave like "media actors", therefore more "television" inclined to assertiveness, controversy or declaration effective (even to the detriment of clarity of information) often for the mere purpose of increasing the audience. Inevitably, this phenomenon has led to a further exacerbated level of conflict. To this end, Nucci and Scaglioni (2022) spoke of "iatrodemia", that is, an epidemic of doctors on TV: "throwing themselves into the arena among polemicists, dwarfs and dancers, they brought medicine into the arena of opinions. The problem is that science is not an opinion. And that this perception changes our way of considering risk and disease" (11). According to the authors, the result is the loss of doctors' authority, in favour of the strengthening of anti-scientific thinking, precisely at a time when trust in the medical establishment would be crucial. In fact, they argue that, from the early stages of the pandemic, on the one hand we have witnessed to the depoliticisation of healthcare decisions, presented as "technical" choices dictated by "experts", therefore indisputable; on the other hand, to the politicisation of doctors, who at the first divergent opinions have become the main bearers of this or that battle. Thus, the authors conclude, to date we have doctors ubiquitous on TV, who now also give clear signs of political affiliation. These phenomena have done nothing but exacerbate a more general feeling that current Western society is going through a crisis of skills, a crisis of legitimacy of scientific knowledge, as postmodern thought had theorised since the 1990s. This trend is enforced by the phenomenon of the prêt-à-porter or passe-partout scientist. In fact, more and more and above all in the natural, physical, mathematical and even medical sciences, scientists publicly express their opinions about areas that go beyond their specific area of expertise. And if a physicist (rather than an epidemiologist) starts talking about virus predictions; a virologist (and not a GP or a hospital doctor) about anti-COVID patients and therapies; a pharmacologist, a virologist, a physicist, an immunologist, a biochemist or molecular biologist (and not an agronomist) about biodynamic agriculture; a biologist or a neurologist (and not a psychologist or a sociologist) about what goes through the mind of a no-vax, they all could indirectly and unknowingly convey the tacit message that skills and expertise are not considered fundamental by scientists themselves and that everyone can try their hand at topics that are different from their object of study. This phenomenon now reappears in ways similar to each new theme that conquers the agenda setting. Once, it was sociologists who were accused of talking about everything; now, the role of the know-it-all is slowly being assumed by physicists and mathematicians (Carlo Rovelli & Piergiorgio Odifreddi) who express themselves on everything. Including the war in Ukraine. Hence, as Gobo & Campo (2021) already stated, the crisis of skills and legitimacy of knowledge seems to be not only the product of forces external to science but also of scientists themselves.

Works cited

3M (2021). *State of Science Index* 2021. https://multimedia.3m.com/mws/media/20192600/3m-2021-sosi-global-report.pdf (11 February 2025).

Achterberg, P., de Koster, W. & van der Waal, J. (2017). A science confidence gap: Education, trust in scientific methods, and trust in scientific institutions in the United States, 2014. *Public Understanding of Science*, 26, 6, 704–720. doi: 10.1177/0963662515617367.

Bucchi, M. (2008). Dal deficit al dialogo, dal dialogo alla partecipazione – e poi? Modelli di interazione tra scienza e pubblico. *Rassegna Italiana di Sociologia*, 49, 3, 377–402.

Bucchi, M. (2021). Per aumentare le vaccinazioni investiamo in fiducia. *Nature Italy*. https://www.nature.com/articles/d43978-021-00004-x (11 February 2025).

Bucchi, M. & Neresini, F. (2002). Biotech remains unloved by the more informed. *Nature*, 416, 261. doi.org/10.1038/416261a.

Bucchi, M. & Neresini, F. (2008). Science and Public Participation. In E.J. Hackett, O. Amsterdamska, M. Lynch & J. Wajcman (eds.), *The Handbook of Science and Technology Studies* (pp. 449–72). Cambridge, London: The MIT Press.

Bucchi, M. & Trench, B. (2017). Science Communication and Science in Society: A Conceptual Review in Ten Keywords. *TECNOSCIENZA: Italian Journal of Science & Technology Studies*, 7, 2, 151–168.

Campo, E., Gobo, G., Galeotti, M. & Parra Saiani, P. (2021). Limiti e fallimenti dei modelli epidemiologici e previsionali nell'epidemia di SARS-COV-2. In A. Favretto, A. Maturo & S. Tomelleri (eds.), *L'impatto Sociale del Covid-19* (pp. 39–48). Milano: Franco Angeli.

Cinelli, M., Quattrociocchi, W., Galeazzi, A., Valensise, C.M., Brugnoli, E., Schmidt, A.L., Zola, P., Zollo, F. & Scala, A. (2020). The COVID-19 social media infodemica. *Scientific Reports*, 10, 16598. doi: 10.1038/s41598-020-73510-5.

Collins, H.M. & Evans, R. (2002). The Third Wave of Science Studies: Studies of Expertise and Experience. *Social Studies of Science*, 32, 2, 235–296. doi.org/10.1177/0306312702032002.

Converse, P.E. (1964). The nature of belief systems in mass publics. In D.E. Apter (ed.), *Ideology and Its Discontent* (pp. 206–261). New York: Free Press of Glencoe.

Converse, P.E. (1970). Attitudes and Non-attitudes: Continuation of a dialogue. In E.R. Tufte (ed.), *The Quantitative Analysis of Social Problems* (pp. 168–189). Boston: Addison-Wesley.

Epstein, S. (1995). The Construction of Lay Expertise: AIDS Activism and the Forging of Credibility in the Reform of Clinical Trials. *Science, Technology, & Human Values*, 20, 4, 408–437. doi.org/10.1177/016224399502000402.

Eyal, G. (2019). *The Crisis of Expertise*. Cambridge: Polity Press.

Fahy, D. & Lewenstein, B. (2014). Scientists in Popular Culture: The Making of Celebrities. In M. Bucchi & B. Trench (eds.), *Routledge Handbook of Public Communication of Science and Technology* (pp. 83–96). London, New York: Routledge.

Feyerabend, P.K. (1979). *Contro il metodo*. Milano: Feltrinelli.

Fleck, L. (1986). The Problem of Epistemology. In R.S. Cohen & T. Schnelle (eds.), *Cognition and Fact: Materials on Ludwik Fleck* (pp. 79–112). Dordrecht: Springer Netherlands.

Fletcher, R., Kalogeropoulos, A., Simon, F.M. et al. (2020). *Information inequality in the UK coronavirus communications crisis*. Reuters Institute report. Reuters Institute for the Study of Journalism, Oxford. https://reutersinstitute.politics.ox.ac.uk/information-inequality-uk-coronavirus-communications-crisis (11 February 2025).

Franck, G. (2014). Économie de l'attention. In Y. Citton (ed.), *L'économie de l'attention: Nouvel horizon du capitalisme?* (pp. 55–72). Paris: La Découverte.

Garfinkel, H. (1967). *Studies in Ethnomethodology*. Englewood Cliffs, New Jersey: Prentice-Hall.

Gazendam, A., Ekhtiari, S., Wong, E., Madden, K., Naji, L., Phillips, M., Mundi, R., Bhandari, M. & Mohit, M. (2020). The "Infodemic" of Journal Publication Associated with the Novel Coronavirus Disease. *The Journal of Bone and Joint Surgery*, 102, 13, e64.

Gobo, G. & Campo, E. (2021). Covid-19 in Italy: should sociology matter? *The European Sociologist*, 46, 12.

Gobo, G. & Marcheselli, V. (2022). *Science, Technology and Society: An Introduction*, London: Palgrave Macmillan.

Gobo, G. & Sena, B. (2022). Questioning and disputing vaccination policies. Scientists and experts in the Italian public debate. *Bulletin of Science, Technology & Society*, 42, 1/2, 25–38. doi.org/10.1177/02704676221080928.

Gray, J., Bounegru, L. & Venturini, T. (2020). 'Fake news' as infrastructural uncanny. *New media & Society*, 22, 2, 317–341. doi.org/10.1177/1461444819856912.

Habgood-Coote, J. (2019). Stop Talking about Fake News! *Inquiry* 62, 9–10, 1033–65. doi.org/10.1080/0020174X.2018.1508363.

Harding, S. (1986). *The Science Question in Feminism.* Ithaca (NY) e London: Cornell University Press.

Hornsey, M.J., Lobera, J. & Díaz-Catalán, C. (2020). Vaccine hesitancy is strongly associated with distrust of conventional medicine, and only weakly associated with trust in alternative medicine. *Social Science & Medicine*, 255, 113019. doi: 10.1016/j.socscimed.2020.113019.

Jasanoff, S. (2005). *Designs on Nature: Science and Democracy in Europe and the United States.* Princeton: Princeton University Press.

Krosnick, J.A., & Abelson, R.P. (1992). The case for measuring attitude strength in surveys. In J.M. Tanur (ed.), *Questions about questions: Inquiries into the cognitive bases of surveys* (pp. 177–203). New York: Russell Sage Foundation.

Kuhn, T.S. (1962). *La struttura delle rivoluzioni scientifiche.* Torino: Einaudi.

Lello, E. (2020). Populismo anti-scientifico o nodi irrisolti della biomedicina? Prospettive a confronto intorno al movimento free vax. *Rassegna Italiana di Sociologia*, 3, 479–508. doi: 10.1423/98558.

Moran, P. (2020). Social Media: A Pandemic of Misinformation. *The American Journal of Medicine*, 133, 11, 1247–1248. doi: 10.1016/j.amjmed.2020.05.021.

Newman, N, Fletcher, R. & Schulz, A, et al. (2021). Digital news report 2021. Digital news report, Reuters Institute for the Study of Journalism, Oxford. https://reutersinstitute.politics.ox.ac.uk/digital-news-report/2021 (11 February 2025).

Nichols, T. (2017). *The Death of Expertise: The Campaign Against Established Knowledge and Why It Matters.* Oxford University Press.

Nielsen, R.K., Fletcher, R., Newman, N. et al. (2020). Navigating the 'infodemic': how people in six countries access and rate news and information about coronavirus. Reuters Institute report, Reuters Institute for the Study of Journalism, Oxford. https://reutersinstitute.politics.ox.ac.uk/infodemic-how-people-six-countries-access-and-rate-news-and-information-about-coronavirus (11 February 2025).

Nielsen, R.K, Schulz, A. & Fletcher, L. (2021). An ongoing infodemic: how people in eight countries access news and information about coronavirus a year into the pandemic. Reuters Institute report, Reuters Institute for the Study of Journalism, Oxford. https://reutersinstitute.politics.ox.ac.uk/ongoing-infodemic-how-people-eight-countries-access-news-and-information-about-coronavirus-year (11 February 2025).

Nucci, P. & Scaglioni, M. (2022). *Iatrodemia. Vizi e virtù dei medici in TV.* Milano: Piemme.

OMS, Novel Coronavirus (2019-nCoV) Situation Report-13, published 2 February 2020.

Papapicco, C. (2020). Informative Contagion: The Coronavirus (COVID-19) in Italian journalism. *Online Journal of Communication and Media Technologies*, 10, 3, e202014. doi.org/10.29333/ojcmt/7938.

Pew Research Center (2020). Science and Scientists Held in High Esteem Across Global Publics. Report. https://www.pewresearch.org/science/wp-content/uploads/sites/16/2020/09/PS_2020.09.29_global-science_REPORT.pdf by Cary Funk, Alec Tyson, Brian Kennedy and Courtney Johnson (11 February 2025).

Popper, K. (2009). *Poscritto alla logica della scoperta scientifica. Il realismo e lo scopo della scienza.* Milano: il Saggiatore.

Putnam, H. (1992). *Renewing Philosophy.* Cambridge: Harvard University Press.

Rothkopf, D.J. (2003). When the Buzz Bites Back. *Washington Post,* 11, 05.

Schäfer, M.S. (2016). Digital Public Sphere. In G. Mazzoleni (ed.), *The International Encyclopedia of Political Communication* (pp. 322–328). Malden (MA): Wiley Blackwell.

Serafini, L. (2021). Infodemia o interesse pubblico? I giornali italiani e la semplificazione dei messaggi sul Covid-19. *Cultura & Comunicazione*, 11,18, 30–35.

Shafir, E., Simonson, I. &Tversky, A. (1993). Reason-based choice. *Cognition*, 49, 114–42. doi: 10.1016/0010-0277(93)90034-s.

Shapin, S. (1988). The House of Experiment in Seventeenth-Century England. *Isis*, 79, 3, 373–404. doi.org/10.1086/354773.

Sigma Consulting (2020). Osservatorio Sociale sugli Orientamenti dei Marchigiani. Opinioni e stati d'animo dei marchigiani al tempo del coronavirus. https://www.sigmaconsulting.biz/blog/post/opinioni-e-stati-danimo-dei-marchigiani-al-tempo-del-coronavirus (11 February 2025).

Simon, F.M., & Camargo, C.Q. (2023). Autopsy of a metaphor: The origins, use and blind spots of the 'infodemic'. *New Media & Society*, *25*, 8, 2219–2240. doi.org/10.1177/14614448211031.

Sudman, S., Bradburn, N.M. & Schwarz, N. (1996). *Thinking about answers: The application of cognitive processes to survey methodology.* San Francisco: Jossey-Bass.

Todorov, T. (2001). *Imperfect Garden: The Legacy of Humanism*, Princeton: Princeton University Press.

Zarocostas, J. (2020). How to fight an infodemic. *The Lancet*, 395, 10225. doi: 10.1016/S0140-6736(20)30461-X.

Enrico Campo / Luca Serafini

COVID-19, Mass Media, and Science Communication: The Case of Conflicts between Scientists in Italy

Abstract

The communicative phenomena connected to the massive media coverage of scientific knowledge during the COVID-19 pandemic have often been analysed in the public and academic debate by using terms of an immediate impact like "fake news" and "infodemic". However, rather than look at the simple dissemination of (supposedly) unfounded or pseudoscientific news, we believe it is more profitable to shift our attention to the intertwining of the scientific and media spheres. The objective of our contribution is thus to reconstruct this intertwining through an analysis of two of the major conflicts that affected the Italian public debate during the first wave of the pandemic. Our hypothesis is that the situation of uncertainty and conflict in the interpretation of certain phenomena related to the circulation of the virus was not generated only or even primarily by the spread of false news, but was instead the result of a spiral dynamic that affected the multiple logics behind the functioning of the media, the scientific community, civil society, and politics. To explore this hypothesis, we will discuss the main factors that influence scientific communication in the media and then discuss the conflicts between scientists in particular. The third and fourth sections are instead dedicated to the reconstruction of the two conflicts that are the objects of our analysis, that is the debates around the contagiousness of asymptomatic carriers of the virus and the alleged loss of potency of the virus. To this end, 819 articles were selected which include both interviews released by a list of the fifty best-known experts in Italy, and articles in which the statements provided in other contexts were reported (primarily in television interviews) and published in the primary Italian newspapers and information websites.

Keywords: COVID-19, scientists, conflicts, mass media.

Enrico Campo, University of Milan, ORCID: 0000-0002-3875-7880.
Luca Serafini, University of Florence, ORCID: 0000-0002-5425-161X.

1. Introduction

The communicative phenomena connected to the massive and essential media coverage of knowledge and scientific discoveries made during the COVID-19 pandemic have often been analysed in the public and academic debate by using terms of an immediate impact. Expressions like "fake news," "post-truth," "pseudoscience," and "infodemic" (Rothkopf, 2003), already used prior to the pandemic, have had particular success during this period. Thanks to their icasticity, these terms are able to effectively represent the idea of an "information virus" said to be spreading uncontrollably due to the media, thereby causing a wave of disinformation about COVID-19. As affirmed by the director general of the World Health Organization Tedros Adhanom Ghebreyesus: "We're not just fighting an epidemic; we're fighting an infodemic" (WHO 2020; Zarocostas, 2020, 676).

The accusations levelled at the media are not without foundation: Italian newspapers, in particular through their social media pages, have repeatedly resorted to headlines that, in many cases, greatly simplified information of a scientific nature that the articles they referred to sought to convey, at times going so far as to completely distort their message (Serafini, 2021). More generally, media narratives of the contagion have underlined a high level of both spectacle and contradiction (Pedroni, 2020), contributing, in part, to disorienting the public. In terms of receiving information, the model that has operated as an implicit reference point is the so-called "deficit model," which identifies public ignorance as the cause of false and pseudoscientific news. However, as has been highlighted by several studies, the same stark contrast between "true" and "false" news or between science and pseudoscience greatly simplifies a much more complex situation (Gordin, 2017; Habgood-Coote, 2019). The notion of an infodemic for example, tends to enclose a variety of very different communicative phenomena within an easy-to-understand umbrella term (Simon & Camargo, 2021) that simplistically attributes the entire responsibility of communicative distortions that took place during the pandemic to the mass media. Rather than looking at the simple dissemination of (allegedly) unfounded or pseudoscientific news, we believe it is more profitable to shift our attention to the intertwining of the scientific and media spheres. The objective of our contribution is to reconstruct this intertwining through an analysis of two of the major conflicts that affected the Italian public debate during the first wave of the pandemic, that is, from January to June 2020. Our hypothesis is that the situation of uncertainty was not generated solely or even primarily by the dissemination of false news but was instead the result of a spiral dynamic that affected the multiple logics behind the functioning of the media, the scientific community, civil society, and politics. To explore this hypothesis, we will briefly review the main factors that influence scientific communication in the media in the next section and then, in the following section, discuss the conflicts between scientists in particular. The third and fourth sections are instead dedicated to the reconstruction of the two conflicts that are the objects of our analysis.

2. Scientists and the Mass Media

The problem of communicating scientific content to a wide audience is certainly not new. Indeed, the difficulty of scientific dissemination and the associated public visibility of some scientists are as old as modern science. As such, if scientists have always had a role in public culture, it is also true that the pandemic produced some substantially new conditions or exacerbated some trends that were already visible previously. Thus, rather than looking at the simple dissemination of unfounded or pseudoscientific information, it seems to us more interesting to shift attention to the dynamics within the scientific community as they manifested themselves in the media.

As a consequence, for a better understanding of the problems encountered by scientific communication during the pandemic, the following aspects should at last be kept in mind:

- The public to which scientific communication is addressed is not unitary and monolithic; rather, audiences are multiple and heterogeneous in terms of their cognitive abilities, cultural interests, levels of education, as well as their interest in science (Bucchi, 2008); therefore communication should, in principle, be modulated with respect to these dimensions. Yet, the pandemic – and its countermeasures – concerned a vast audience, thus making it much more difficult to communicate with a certain level of detail.
- The contents of communication. Knowledge about the virus itself and the disease it caused was new, necessarily uncertain, and ever-changing, unlike other situations in which knowledge is stable and generally accepted. As a result, in this uncertain context, the simultaneous presence of a plurality of experts and skills was necessary.
- Media formats obviously condition the ways in which content is transmitted and discursive spaces are often quite reduced, compressed, and contingent; they are thus inadequate for tackling very complex topics whose content is constantly evolving.
- Media visibility. While the public visibility of some scientists is not a new phenomenon, the pandemic gave the scientific community unprecedented media exposure. In this context, the spectacularisation processes of science were greatly accelerated and some scientists effectively became media actors and true celebrities (Fahy & Lewenstein, 2014; Franck, 2019).

3. Conflicts between experts

Controversies and conflicts (including personal ones) between scientists are constitutive of the scientific process even in situations of "normal science" (Kuhn, 1962). On the one hand then, during the pandemic the media illuminated the "normal" face of science, that is, an entirely "human" and "social" enterprise made up of conflicts, interests, different opinions, and certainties being called into question after a few weeks. On the other hand, the factors mentioned above and the general hyper-mediatisation of scientific knowledge that took place during the pandemic contributed to exacerbating these same conflicts.

However, responsibility cannot be entirely attributed to the media system. The scientists themselves in fact contributed to conveying a flawed image of their diatribes. It is particularly significant, for example, that scientists in conflict have at times – as we will better see below – interpreted opposing positions to their own as unscientific or not adhering to "facts" or have presented the results of ongoing research and uncertain data as if they were well sedimented. This has probably contributed to clouding the constructive nature of the scientific debate. In short, some scientists have represented the normal discussions that always play a role in scientific progress (especially in a situation of marked cognitive uncertainty such as that caused by a new and unknown virus) as a diatribe between science and pseudoscience and have appealed to their colleagues to stick to "the facts" rather than just providing opinions.

Furthermore, precisely because of the media exposure, the interpretative conflict we witnessed was only externally linked to individual personalities, while at times it was articulated as a conflict between individual disciplines with reciprocal accusations of incompetence on a disciplinary basis. In particular, with reference to the material we have collected, during the pandemic two types of conflicts emerged within the scientific community: intra-disciplinary, in which scientists belonging to the same discipline clashed over the interpretation of specific data or on the effectiveness of a certain policy; and inter-disciplinary, which concerned scientists belonging to different disciplines. This type of conflict concerned not only the interpretation of data but also doubts about one's relative competence.

Finally, the conflict was further exasperated by the fact that scientists were not only consulted by the mass media as communicators or simple *specialists* in a discipline, but were also called upon to provide practical and political (and therefore not only scientific) advice. In so doing scientists often went beyond their own field of inquiry by providing responses beyond their specific expertise.

Let us now examine in further detail how these conflicts were articulated in relation to two topics, namely the debate surrounding the contagiousness of asymptomatic individuals and on the presumed loss of strength of the virus over time, which we have subjected to scrutiny through research gathered from newspapers and news sites from 01 January to 30 November 2020. To this end, 819 articles were selected which include both interviews released by a list of the fifty best-known experts at the national level as well as articles in which statements provided in other contexts were reported (mainly television interviews) and published in the major newspapers and online (*Corriere della Sera*, *Repubblica*, *Tg Com24*, *Il Messaggero*, *Il Fatto Quotidiano*, *Fanpage*, *La Stampa*, *Il Giornale*, *Il Sole 24 ore*, *TPI*, *Open*).[1]

4. Asymptomatic Individuals: contagiousness, viral load, and tracking

Asymptomatic individuals – that is, those who contracted the virus without manifesting symptoms of the disease – were the subject of debate during all stages of the infection. Experts were asked to determine whether or not asymptomatic carriers of the virus were able to transmit infection, or whether it was spread only by people who exhibited symptoms of the disease. This was clearly a relevant issue since it concerned various *lockdown policies*. The conflict between experts had already begun to emerge in the first few months of 2020: a study published in *The Lancet* (Chan et al., 2020) in January 2020 highlighted the possibility of infection being transmitted even by asymptomatic individuals. This was joined by a study which presented similar conclusions published in the *New England Journal of Medicine* in February (Rothe et al., 2020). The two studies led scientists such as virologist Roberto Burioni, immunologist Guido Silvestri, paediatrician and infectious disease specialist Susanna Esposito, virologist Ilaria Capua and others to talk about contagion being transmitted by asymptomatic individuals in terms that were at times probabilistic and at times of absolute certainty, using expressions like "without a shadow of a doubt."[2] However, such certainties were not shared by other scientists: after the case of two Chinese tourists testing positive in Rome on 30 January 2020, Giuseppe Ippolito, infectious disease specialist and scientific director of the Spallanzani Institute, reassured the population with the following words: "Citizens can rest assured because the real risk of transmission occurs through symptomatic individuals."[3] Similar

1 Publications were selected on the basis of both their daily circulation and the online traffic of their respective websites and social pages. The NVivo10 text analysis programme was used for data organization and analysis.

2 "Roberto Burioni, Lo studio choc: coronavirus replica bene anche in chi non ha sintomi" (23 February 2020), *Il Tempo*, https://bit.ly/36LSW6m.

3 Adalgisa Marrocco, "La psicosi da Coronavirus in Italia è ingiustificata: il rischio contagio è improbabile" (31 January 2020), *Huffington Post*, https://bit.ly/3wKACVQ.

positions, between February and March 2020, were taken by other scientists such as the hygienist and toxicologist Fabrizio Pregliasco ("it's difficult for an asymptomatic subject to significantly infect another person"[4]) and the infectious disease specialist Paolo Grossi ("based on current scientific knowledge, their level of contagiousness is minimal"[5]). The clash began in June 2020, coinciding with debate on the supposed attenuation of the viral load of the virus – which we will discuss in further detail in the next section. At least three different positions emerged over the course of the summer.

The first position, that can be summarised by the formula "a COVID-positive person is not a sick person," was that of those who expressed themselves with certainty about the non-contagiousness of asymptomatic individuals. It made reference to the "document" titled "SARS-CoV-2 in Italy today and Covid-19"[6] which was signed by 10 scientists from different disciplines who argued that we were facing an exponential increase in "weakly-positive" individuals who were consequently non-contagious. The other cornerstone on this front was the June 2020 study by the Mario Negri Institute, the results of which were disseminated in the media by the director of the institute, nephrologist Giuseppe Remuzzi, who also highlighted a low viral load in asymptomatic subjects (in his institute) and maintained its non-contagiousness.[7]

This study, however, was strongly contested by other scientists: a counter-document signed by seven experts from different disciplines stated, among other things, that it was not proved that "the virus isolated in subjects who have been asymptomatic for several days has no infectious capacity in vitro."[8] Other experts, from the hygienist and epidemiologist Paolo Bonanni to the pulmonologist Sergio Harari, affirmed that Negri's study was too limited to be able to generalise

4 "Coronavirus: cosa vuol dire essere positivo?" (9 March 2020), *San Donato Group*, https://bit.ly/3D8Pb73.

5 Simona Ravizza, "Coronavirus Lombardia, Malati emersi e numero di tamponi: ecco che cosa influenza la curva" (27 March 2020), *Corriere della Sera*, https://bit.ly/36usxdo.

6 In truth, it was a short post on Facebook and published in the *Journal* on June 24, without any scientific references, signed by Alberto Zangrillo, Matteo Bassetti, Massimo Clementi, Donato Greco, Giorgio Palù, Giuseppe Remuzzi, Roberto Rigoldi, the microbiologist Arnaldo Caruso, the anesthetists and resuscitators Luciano Gattinoni and Luca Lorini. See Valerio Berra, "'In Italia ormai è raro il ricovero per Coronavirus, impennata di debolmente positivi' – Il documento firmato da 10 scienziati" (23 June 2020), Open, https://bit.ly/3NyfzMz.

7 Marco Imarisio, "Coronavirus, Remuzzi: 'I nuovi positivi non sono contagiosi, stop alla paura'" 19 June 2020, *Corriere della Sera*, https://bit.ly/36rM6mB.

8 Signatories of the document were infectious disease specialists Marcello Tavio, Massimo Andreoni, Giovanni Di Perri, Massimo Galli and Claudio Maria Mastroianni as well as virologist and microbiologist Carlo Federico Perno. Margherita De Bac, "Virus poco contagioso? 'C'è ed è molto pericoloso. Non è diverso da quello in Brasile'" (28 June 2020), *Corriere della Sera*, https://bit.ly/3wAIBVF.

the results.[9] This second front, which we could define as "uncertain," maintained that it was not possible to express the contagiousness of asymptomatic individuals with certainty either in one sense or another.

The third position instead was represented by those who continued to maintain a position of certainty on the contagiousness of asymptomatic patients: among these we can include microbiologist, parasitologist, and expert on tropical diseases Andrea Crisanti, who repeatedly referred to evidence from the study conducted to Vo' Euganeo (later published in *Nature*) as proof of the contagiousness of asymptomatic individuals, expressing himself in a caustic manner towards those who sustained opposing theses ("When they tell me asymptomatic people don't transmit infection, I throw up my hands"[10]). Even physicist and expert in computational epidemiology Alessandro Vespignani discredited the theses of those who argued for the non-contagiousness of asymptomatic individuals in numerous articles with phrases like "the asymptomatic and pre-symptomatic are contagious and must be traced, otherwise we might as well put a blindfold on and pray to God."[11]

However, it should be noted that even within the first group the positions were not unequivocal. Infectious disease specialist Matteo Bassetti repeatedly supported the need to distinguish three types of asymptomatic patients according to their viral load and to calculate with laboratory experiments the viral load below which one could be considered no longer contagious.[12] This was a position rejected by the anaesthetist Alberto Zangrillo, according to whom "trying to calculate the standard viral load below which you are not contagious is a useless exercise, simply because the viral loads in circulation are unable to cause infection."[13]

Further confusion on the issue was generated by the positions taken by the WHO, which provided different opinions on at least three separate occasions: in February 2020 ("transmission by asymptomatic individuals is relatively rare" read one of its reports); in March 2020 ("patients emit more viruses in the early stages of the disease, even when they are pre-symptomatic"); and in June 2020, when the infectious disease specialist Maria Van Kerkhove, head of the WHO

9 Cristina Marrone, "Coronavirus, i positivi sono meno infettivi? Il dibattito tra gli esperti" (20 June 2020), *Corriere della Sera*, https://bit.ly/3uw65Zg.

10 "Crisanti: Asintomatici non contagiosi? Mi cascano le braccia" (25 June 2020), *Adnkronos*, https://bit.ly/3JGQ7C5.

11 Paolo Giordano, Alessandro Vespignani, "Covid, 7 principi razionali per affrontare il contagio" (02 November 2020), *Corriere della Sera*, https://bit.ly/36mqmbX.

12 "L'Oms: 'E' molto raro che una persona asintomatica possa trasmettere il coronavirus.' L'infettivologo Bassetti: 'Cautela, esistono diverse tipologie'" (09 June 2020), *La Stampa*, https://bit.ly/3iz5EYL.

13 "Alberto Zangrillo, la polemica tra virologi: 'Un esercizio inutile', perché la carica virale non è preoccupante" (20 June 2020), *Libero*, https://bit.ly/3IDnEf1.

anti-COVID-19 technical team, stated: “It is very rare that an asymptomatic person can transmit the coronavirus,” only to correct herself and mention “limited datasets.” This gave rise to an “international” conflict which also involved Italian experts. Among these, the doctor and expert in Evidence-Based Medicine (based on a statistical approach) Nino Cartabellotta stigmatised the behaviour of “a representative from the highest international health authority” who launched into “bold and dangerous statements”. The same hygienist, Walter Ricciardi, a member of the WHO, commenting on the statements of Van Kerkhove stated “it is precisely the transmission from asymptomatic or rather paucisymptomatic or pre-symptomatic that differentiates it [SARS-CoV-2] from Sars and Mers. In a month it has spread all over the world while in other pandemics it takes 6 months to a year.”[14]

Thus, the conflict began on this issue in the early stages of the pandemic and continued, involving experts from different disciplines, over a protracted period of time and was both intra-disciplinary and inter-disciplinary in nature. It should also be noted that even after the summer of 2020 an interpretative conflict persisted between various experts, including virologist Giorgio Palù and the aforementioned Bassetti, who, in the autumn of 2020 during the second wave, reiterated the non-dangerousness and the non-contagiousness of asymptomatic individuals.[15] Finally, it should also be noted that many experts changed position over time: among the many possible examples we can mention Fabrizio Pregliasco, the infectious disease specialist and epidemiologist Donato Greco (who supported the thesis of the contagiousness of asymptomatic patients[16] between March and May but subsequently supported the document “SARS-CoV-2 in Italy today and COVID-19”), and the hygienist Pierluigi Lopalco (who in June 2020 contested the WHO statements about the low contagiousness of asymptomatic patients only to express himself in these terms two months later: “the bogeyman of asymptomatic people who plague the world should be revised a little”).[17]

14 Cristina Marrone, “Gli asintomatici sono contagiosi? Ecco cosa dice la scienza” (10 June 2020), *Corriere della Sera*, https://bit.ly/3wDpWsk.

15 Valentina Dardari, “‘Il 96% asintomatico’, ‘Falso’: ora è scontro tra i virologi” (24 October 2020), *il Giornale*, https://bit.ly/3Nxmju2.

16 Donato Greco, “Sorvegliare e pulire: eccessi da sanificazione” (19 May 2020,) *Scienza in rete*, https://bit.ly/3IDpxID.

17 Public page of Pier Luigi Lopalco, *Facebook:* https://bit.ly/3IVCNsn (19 May 2020).

5. The "clinically dead virus"

One of the most heated conflicts developed around the well-known phrase pronounced by Alberto Zangrillo on 31 May 2020, during a television broadcast: "the virus from a clinical point of view no longer exists." In support of this thesis, Zangrillo referenced a study by virologist Massimo Clementi and statements by Guido Silvestri. In truth, his statement did not indicate the virus was gone, but signalled evidence that no one disputed: a large reduction in hospitalisations and ICU admissions. As for how to interpret this evidence - which was the real bone of contention - various elements were discussed that had previously been the subject of debate (and would continue to be so): contagion by asymptomatic individuals, mutations of the virus, the viral load detected in patients, the lethality of the virus, the role of the climate, the seasonality of the disease and eventual "waves", the effectiveness of drugs and protection measures, the role of containment measures, interaction between the virus and the host.

The idea that the virus had weakened had already circulated around 6 May, following an interview given by Clementi to *Corriere della Sera*, in which he cited the study he was participating in, together with many Italian hospitals, and whose goal was to "have constant monitoring of the sequences of the virus": the expected result of the study was to show that "this new coronavirus may slowly become harmless, like its "cousins", which are responsible for colds."[18] Still, many had already claimed, even if only in terms of a possibility, that the virus was losing strength (without commenting on possible causes). In fact, between mid-April and early May, hospital radiologist Maurizio Borghetti, immunologist Francesco Le Foche, epidemiologist Massimo Ciccozzi and the aforementioned Palù and Bassetti expressed themselves in this sense. During the month of May 2020, interest in the topic increased progressively, also and primarily because on 4th May, restrictive measures were eased in Italy (the so-called "phase 2") and, despite the expectation of a resurgence of infections and hospitalisations, these continued to decline. For some, this was evidence that the virus had mutated, that the viral load had decreased, or that the disease had changed, which might then die out naturally. For others, however, the decline in hospitalisations was simply due to a reduction in the number of infected persons.

At least in the initial phase, opened by Zangrillo's famous phrase, the clash seemed to concern a different approach to the epidemic: the clinicians (who worked, directly or indirectly, in the hospital in close contact with patients) supported the thesis of the "clinically dead virus" while those who relied on an approach more closely linked to epidemiological models of viral spread con-

18 Laura Cuppini, "Il coronavirus sta davvero perdendo potenza? Ecco cosa sappiamo oggi" (06 May 2020), *Corriere della Sera*, https://bit.ly/37PsngT.

tested it. Already by 13th May, when the conflict had yet to assume the harsh tones it would take on later, Clementi explained the difference in perspective with respect to his colleagues who arrived at conclusions different from his own: "they start with algorithms, with initial assumptions, with amazing big data, with pre-established keys of interpretation. [But then] they find themselves in front of the clinical reality […] irrefutable! – and the whole castle falls down."[19] Thus, also Zangrillo, again in the aforementioned interview, affirmed "there is only one number that is valid" and "it is the evidence: in this country we heard a professor from Boston a month ago, who is an epidemiologist-statistician named Vespignani, who influenced the government's choices by saying that 151 thousand intensive care units had to be built." In fact, Zangrillo here seemed to confuse Vespignani with mathematician Stefano Merler, who was responsible for the epidemiological model that was to be the basis upon which the government designed and adopted measures for the so-called phase two (Campo et al., 2021). Yet, the reference did not seem accidental, given that, in an interview about a month earlier, Vespignani defended his approach in this way: "I'm not good at disassembling the motor of a virus, finding a vaccine, but I work with data to understand how many infected there will be tomorrow, in a month, in Milan, Bergamo, or New York […] [there is a] difference between a virus mechanic and an epidemiologist." And so then "virologists – as I will explain – might be luminaries, but sometimes they are the least suitable people for understanding how epidemics develop."[20]

At the same time, the conflict about the clinical death of the virus crossed disciplinary boundaries and some scientists changed their minds or diluted their position over time. The most significant in this sense was certainly Clementi, who, only 15 days before publicly supporting the thesis that the virus was losing strength, said in a television interview that SARS-CoV-2 "seems relatively stable compared to the others [Coronavirus]."[21]

Clearly, the debate was closely linked to the policies governing the circulation of the virus that were about to be adopted, which is why it acquired enormous relevance and visibility in the media. In the most intense phase of the clash, in the period from June to July 2020, experts were often asked to take sides for or against the hypothesis that the virus was losing strength. In one of the phases of

19 Luca Telese, "Clementi a TPI: 'Il virus non è più aggressivo, è un dato di fatto. Ma certi altri virologi ragionano con gli algoritmi'" (13 May 2020), *The International Post,* https://bit.ly/3IEPZl6.

20 Luca Telese, "Vespignani a TPI: 'I virologi italiani non hanno capito nulla, per sconfiggere il virus servono le 3T'" (03 May 2020), *The Post Internazionale,* https://bit.ly/3JJu79x. Then, on 21st May, he labeled the hypothesis that the virus was getting weaker as "bar gossip."

21 "Il virologo Clementi a Tgcom24: 'Il virus non è cambiato durante l'epidemia'" (14 April 2020), *Tgcom 24,* https://www.youtube.com/watch?v=faSne6olJCo.

greatest tension, two groups of scientists took a strong public position on the matter: the first group, which included ten of the most well-known scientists at a public level and from different disciplinary backgrounds, published on social media the aforementioned document of 23 June entitled "SARS-CoV-2 in Italy today and COVID-19," in which it was argued that "hospitalization for symptoms attributable to viral infection is now a rare phenomenon [...]. The virological evidence, in complete parallel, shows a constant increase in cases with a low or very low viral load. Studies are in progress to explain the cause." This group of "optimists" – accused of superficiality by the opposing side – was contrasted by another group of more cautious scientists – accused in turn of "catastrophism" – who published a document a few days later (on 28 June) that responded to "the 10" in which they declared themselves to be "worried that optimistic declarations about the reduced contagiousness of SARS-CoV-2 could cause people to mistakenly believe that the danger had abated. [...] The virus currently circulating is active and contagious," and is "capable of causing extremely serious damage similar to what it did at the beginning of the epidemic."[22] It is interesting to note how the parties involved, especially the representatives of the most extreme positions in the most heated phases, did not see the conflict in terms of a difference in interpretation of data and the phenomena under discussion, but rather as a problem of a lack of scientificity or competence of the opposing side. Appeals to limit oneself to the "real" evidence or the "real" data were levelled at both sides and, in some cases, even led to actual personal attacks.[23]

22 Margherita De Bac, "Virus poco contagioso? 'C'è ed è molto pericoloso. Non è diverso da quello in Brasile'" (28 June 2020), *Corriere della Sera*, https://bit.ly/3wAIBVF.

23 Silvestri (25/5): "I am only pro-science, pro-evidence, and pro-data;" Zangrillo (30/5) "For three months they have been showing us a series of numbers which have zero evidence, which have zero value;" Clementi (25/06): "Crisanti until recently was working with malaria, now he has been catapulted into this problem and I would invite him to be careful because we're not talking about malaria here. Each of us has a story, I've been a virologist for thirty years;" Palù (5/07) "The crux of the discussion, even in science, is the confrontation between peers, between virologists. Certainly not with those who accredit themselves as virologists or are accredited by the media as such" (the reference here was to Crisanti who was accused of being a "mosquito scientist"); Galli (07/10), to Nicola Porro's statement that "yesterday Professor Bassetti told me that 94% are weak positives or asymptomatic," replied "It's a lie, absolutely yes. Bassetti can't say that because he can't know it – continued Galli – He should take a tour in my department to see how things are going, let's not joke around;" Bassetti (11/30) "The other night there was a veterinarian talking about vaccines [...] we need to get our competences straight [...] everyone should keep to what they know" (the reference was to Ilaria Capua).

6. Conclusions

In our opinion, analysis of these two conflicts provides empirical evidence that allows us to further problematise the situation of uncertainty generated by the spread of the pandemic, avoiding the simplifications that reduced distortions in communication exclusively to the dissemination of false news by the media.

As we demonstrated, it was the scientists themselves, in part thanks to the unusual media exposure, who interpreted the normal disputes that take place within their community as conflicts between science and pseudoscience, between indisputable truths and opinions. The absorption of media logic thus led scientists, on the one hand, to assume assertive positions, aimed at demarcating clear boundaries between those who were entitled to express themselves and those who were not (even on a disciplinary basis). However, the same mechanisms also meant that many scientists, as a consequence of their transformation into "media actors," were led to express themselves on issues that were not within their field of expertise.

But this communicative spiral also involved civil society and politics: in fact, a social request for certainty from the sciences was generated which could not be satisfied and which, inevitably, remained unfulfilled. The boundaries between scientific knowledge and political choice were often eroded by the pretence that scientists provide "all-round" solutions, substituting themselves with political decision-makers.

We therefore believe that only by taking the intertwining between different subjects and different communication dynamics into account is it possible to obtain a more complete analytical framework: although the mass media are in certain cases responsible for excessive simplifications or total distortions of scientific knowledge, they do not act as isolated actors. All the interpretations that refer to the diffusion of "fake" news or to the concept of an infodemic tend to convey the idea that it is simple to clearly distinguish between what is true news and what is false. Furthermore, they ultimately entrust to scientists, understood as an indistinct unity, the responsibility of distinguishing the true from the false, where this distinction is more often the subject of dispute. It is therefore incorrect to ignore the role of scientists in fuelling this dynamic, especially when they themselves interpret the conflict in terms of a clash between science and pseudoscience or when they tend to present recent results that have not yet undergone the scrutiny of the scientific community as certainty.

More generally, it is perhaps best to abandon all interpretations based on a single explanatory factor and give up the nostalgic, positivist-flavoured idea that it is easy to distinguish between the truth of facts on the one hand and the falsity of opinions on the other. Especially in "exceptional" situations like a pandemic, it is best not to abandon oneself to the temptation of simplification and, if anything, recognise the complexity of the communication ecosystem.

Works cited

Bucchi, M. (2008). Dal deficit al dialogo, dal dialogo alla partecipazione – e poi? Modelli di interazione tra scienza e pubblico. *Rassegna Italiana di Sociologia*, 3, 377–402.

Campo, E., Gobo, G., Galeotti, M. & Parra Saiani, P. (2021). Limiti e fallimenti dei modelli epidemiologici e previsionali nell'epidemia di SARS-COV-2. In A.R. Favretto, A. Maturo, & S. Tomelleri (eds.), *L'impatto Sociale del Covid-19* (pp. 39–48). Milano: Franco Angeli.

Chan, J. F.-W., Yuan, S., Kok, K.-H., To, K. K.-W., Chu, H., Yang, J., Xing, F., Liu, J., Yip, C. C.-Y., Poon, R. W.-S., Tsoi, H.-W., Lo, S. K.-F., Chan, K.-H., Poon, V. K.-M., Chan, W.-M., Ip, J. D., Cai, J.-P., Cheng, V. C.-C., Chen, H., Yuen, K.-Y. (2020). A familial cluster of pneumonia associated with the 2019 novel coronavirus indicating person-to-person transmission: A study of a family cluster. *The Lancet*, 395(10223), 514–523. https://doi.org/10.1016/S0140-6736(20)30154-9 (20 January 2023).

Fahy, D. & Lewenstein, B. (2014). Scientists in Popular Culture: The Making of Celebrities. In M. Bucchi & B. Trench (eds.), *Routledge Handbook of Public Communication of Science and Technology* (2nd. edition) (pp. 83–96). Abingdon-New York: Routledge.

Franck, G. (2019). The Economy of Attention. *Journal of Sociology*, 1, 8–19. https://doi.org/10.1177/1440783318811778 (10 February 2023).

Gordin, M.D. (2017). "The problem with pseudoscience: Pseudoscience is not the antithesis of professional science but thrives in science's shadow". EMBO Reports, 9, 1482–1485. https://doi.org/10.15252/embr.201744870 (20 July 2022).

Habgood-Coote, J. (2019). "Stop talking about fake news!". *Inquiry*, 9–10, 1033–1065. https://doi.org/10.1080/0020174X.2018.1508363 (12 July 2023).

Kuhn, T. S. (1962). *The Structure of Scientific Revolutions.* Chicago: University of Chicago Press.

Pedroni, M. (2020). Narrazioni virali. Decostruire (e ricostruire) il racconto dell'emergenza coronavirus. *Mediascapes journal*, 15, 24–43.

Rothe, C., Schunk, M., Sothmann, P., Bretzel, G., Froeschl, G., Wallrauch, C., Zimmer, T., Thiel, V., Janke, C., Guggemos, W., Seilmaier, M., Drosten, C., Vollmar, P., Zwirglmaier, K., Zange, S., Wölfel, R. & Hoelscher, M. (2020). Transmission of 2019-nCoV Infection from an Asymptomatic Contact in Germany. *New England Journal of Medicine*, 10, 970–971. https://doi.org/10.1056/NEJMc2001468 (12 February 2023).

Rothkopf, D.J. (2003). When the buzz bites back. *The Washington Post*, 11 May. 07 https://www.washingtonpost.com/archive/opinions/2003/05/11/when-the-buzz-bites-back/bc8cd84f-cab6-4648-bf58-0277261af6cd/ (12 June 2024).

Serafini, L. (2021). Infodemia o interesse pubblico? I giornali italiani e la semplificazione dei messaggi sul Covid-19. *Cultura & Comunicazione*, 18, 30–35.

Simon, F.M. & Camargo, C.Q. (2021). Autopsy of a metaphor: The origins, use and blind spots of the 'infodemic'. *New Media & Society*, 1–22. https://doi.org/10.1177/14614448211031908 (18 January 2023).

WHO: Novel Coronavirus(2019-nCoV)Situation Report-13 (2020). https://www.who.int/docs/default-source/coronaviruse/situation-reports/20200202-sitrep-13-ncov-v3.pdf (10 May 2024).

Zarocostas, J. (2020). How to fight an infodemic. *The Lancet*, 395, 676. https://doi.org/10.1016/S0140-6736(20)30461-X (11 May 2023).

Niccolò Bertuzzi / Elisa Lello

Back to Functionalism? Capturing Language and Pathologising Dissent: from Environmental Movements to Protests against Pandemic Policies

Abstract
This chapter examines how traditional left flagships – such as public health, trust in science and environmental sustainability – have undergone a semantic reversal as neoliberal capitalism has appropriated and repurposed them to legitimise its interests. A systematic reflection on the complex consequences of these semantic reversals in the public sphere and in changing contexts and opportunities for political participation is still lacking. We examine how these processes have intensified in response to the COVID-19 pandemic and the ecological crisis, leading to the stigmatisation of protest movements and the shrinking of the space for political dissent. These semantic reversals, particularly evident in the case of COVID-related protests, allowed for a reproposition of interpretive schemes peculiar to the early days of structural-functionalist literature. This was also possible because these protests were framed as "exceptional": it was precisely the persuasiveness of their discontinuity that justified the abandonment of interpretive tools accumulated over decades by different disciplines. By reading the covid phase not as an exception, but rather as an acceleration of pre-existing dynamics affecting political participation and representation, we recognise in the recovery of functionalist approaches an outcome of justification of existing power relations. By contrast, drawing on qualitative research, we argue for the need for different interpretive perspectives capable of unveiling the ongoing redefinition of the lines of political conflict and contextual processes of re-politicisation.

Keywords: Language capture, public health, sustainability, environmental movements, COVID-19, technocratic governance, greenwashing, functionalism, pathologization of dissent, vaccine hesitancy.

Niccolò Bertuzzi, University of Parma, ORCID: 0000-0003-2929-8931.
Elisa Lello, University of Urbino, ORCID: 0000-0002-5596-5067.

1. Introduction

The central theme that is investigated in this contribution is the process of semantic shift – and, in some cases, overturn – that involves concepts and keywords that traditionally belonged to the field of progressive politics and to "the Left", such as the protection of public health, trust in science, and environmental sustainability. Our main argument is that this process occurred due to a long-standing symbolic and language "capture" by neoliberal capitalism, and accelerated significantly in tandem with the pandemic and the ecological crisis.[1] Thus, while it was relatively easy to identify progressive and regressive positions on these issues until recently, the same keywords have become battlegrounds between (partially) new actors and collective identities at present.

To approach this topic, we can refer to the concept of "green washing" (and to the concept of "ethics washing", which has a similar meaning; as will be demonstrated later, the same discourse should be broadened to include the phenomenon of "participatory washing"). That concept is evoked to allude to strategies whereby some of the industrial sector's objectives are supported via a "painting" of green that makes them appear to be interventions that are aimed at the collective interest. The relevance, as well as the frequency, of occasions and events in which power groups seize Left-wing keywords in this way, only to empty them and bend them to their own particular ends, has a profound effect on the functioning of the public space. This was particularly the case during the recent health crisis (COVID-19 pandemic) and the ecological crisis, which appeared to legitimise and thus accelerate the transition to styles of government marked by the limitation of debate and informational pluralism, as well as by a technocratic process of decision making (Bertuzzi et al., 2022; Shir-Ratz et al., 2022).

However, what is currently lacking is an articulate and systematic reflection on the multiple and complex consequences that these processes have had in the public sphere and on civil society. In the following sections, we will develop a contribution that is aimed at reconstructing the evolutions that have allowed the emergence of such processes of semantic emptying and overturn. We will then focus on the ways in which these processes are changing the context, opportunities and conditions for political participation and protest actions, as well as the perceptions and interpretations thereof, while redefining the geometries of alliances and the lines of political conflict (Lello & Bertuzzi, 2025).

Such analyses and contextualisation shed new light on some important mobilisation experiences during the years 2020 and 2021, thus making it possible to interpret them in a different way from the prevailing interpretation offered by the

1 By this term, we mean not only the climate crisis but also a range of other issues, such as the loss of biodiversity, the exploitation of soil and the alteration of biogeochemical cycles.

media and in the public debate. We propose an emancipatory interpretation because it is emancipated from the colonisation of language and imaginary (Latouche, 2011).

Although this may concern different examples of mobilisations, this chapter, particularly the last part, will focus on the protests that gave expression to the heterogeneous reasons for dissent against the management of the COVID-19 pandemic. We will focus specifically on the Italian case, and will rely on qualitative research investigating the subjective reasons and representations of Italian vaccine-hesitant people[2]. Italy was the first European country to be officially hit by the pandemic in 2020 and was among those most affected, both in terms of the number of victims and regarding the stringency of the measures[3] taken to prevent the spread of the virus.

When examining these protests, both the public discussion and the academic debate demonstrated some reticence to identify within them a demand for participation and an expression of dissent considered worthy of being collected and included in the normal procedures of democratic representation. The stigmatisation of dissent found some justification in the re-propositioning of interpretive schemes peculiar to the early days of structural-functionalist literature on protests and social movements (Le Bon, 1895); according to that perspective, social movements were interpreted via psychologising perspectives that placed more emphasis on the alleged pathological traits of those who protested – called "hysteria" at that time, and currently the conspiracy mentality, ignorance or selfishness – than on their nature as collectives actors moved by (their) reasons and by an underlying rationality (at least a rationality that is internal and based on the existence of structured arguments), by virtue of which social movements can become vectors of social change.

This was also possible because the protests that were related to the pandemic, health policies and vaccines, have been framed as "exceptional", and were consequently interpreted as being different from – and in discontinuity with – the evolutions in social movements, critical citizenship practices and the relationships between grassroots participation, representation and government that were in place prior to the pandemic (Bertuzzi et al., 2022). It is precisely the persuasiveness of such discontinuity and exceptionalism that may, on closer inspection, justify the divestment of interpretive tools that social movement studies had accumulated over decades; however, the same can be said about the established knowledge within the sociology of science and Science and Technology Studies

2 We refer to the concept of Vaccine Hesitancy and Refusal (VHR), as conceptualised by Attwell & Smith (2017).

3 Cfr. The Stringency index compiled by the University of Oxford https://bit.ly/3Kmkukl (12 February 2025).

(STS), which have also been hastily set aside in a public debate that has rushed to surreptitiously retrieve, in the reading of vaccine hesitancy, outdated tools such as the so-called Deficit Model (Simis et al., 2016). This model, which is based on the well-known Bodmer report of 1985, tended to interpret public resistance to particular techno-scientific innovations as merely reflection of ignorance and the inability to understand the scientific method. Nonetheless, STS scholars have been distancing themselves from such simplistic and paternalistic conceptions of the public for decades in order to acknowledge the public's competence, the existence and legitimacy of reasons for doubt or opposition other than ignorance and, above all, the right to have a say in decisions that are intended to have a major impact on the lives of citizens. Based on these arguments, scholars have advocated for the creation of equal channels for discussion between scientists and non-expert citizens, as well as ways of including the latter in the definition of research priorities (Coniglione, 2010).

By contrast, the analysis that we propose does not situate the pandemic situation, particularly the protest demonstrations connected to it, in such an exceptional situation as to require the suspension of the cognitive instruments elaborated over time, but rather places them in full continuity with the changes that have been affecting the main channels of intermediation of social demands between citizens and the political system for decades; that is, political parties, interest and pressure groups, and social movements. The main idea is that what we currently see is the result of changes that have taken shape over decades, and underwent a major acceleration in recent times due to multiple factors , which we will attempt to disentangle. Therefore, in order to interpret what has happened and is happening, it is necessary to move away from a vision that is focused on current events in order to frame them within the changes that have occurred over a longer period.

2. Taking a step back to link current events to the past

As the goal of our work is to discuss how the appropriation of grassroots Leftist battles by neoliberal governance could have occurred, we should begin with what has taken place in the Left during the last few decades. As early as the 1960s, the so-called Silent Revolution, which was brought about by the emergence of so-called post-materialist values (Inglehart, 1977) and the consequent rotation of the Left-Right axis (Kitschelt & McGann, 1995), represented crucial junctures in the gradual distancing of the Centre-Left parties from the working-class perspective and the issues of labour, inequality and redistribution, in order to shift their identities towards cultural and civil rights-oriented claims. While these evolutions occurred in the entire Western European context, the recent history of the Italian Left is particularly emblematic, as it is marked by the presence of the Partito Democratico (PD, Democratic Party) which, since its foundation in 2007, has appropriated the post-communist legacy by combining it with extremely moderate traditions. This, together with choices that have led to organisational models being disconnected from the grassroots level and the territory, and being characterised by the prevalence of mediatisation over organisation, has favoured a particularly sharp and accelerated break with the cultural tradition of the Left and its referents in civil society (Fava, 2013; Floridia, 2019).

Consistent with the perspective of party cartelisation (Katz & Mair, 1995; 2009), the PD has taken part in a course of ideological depolarisation and progressive convergence with parties from the conservative area on the terrain of neoliberalism, at least concerning some key economic policy issues. At the same time, its hegemonic ambitions in the Left field have contributed to the marginalisation and increasing delegitimisation of the actors, both parties and movements, which have arisen to its left (della Porta et al., 2022). The alter-global movements that took to the streets of Genoa in 2001 were already subjected to strong delegitimisation and to the exclusion of their contents and proposals from the public debate (Agnoletto & Guadagnucci, 2011). A similar pattern was repeated in subsequent waves of protest (such as the "Onda Anomala"; Caruso et al., 2010), resulting in a scenario in which alternatives to neoliberalism and austerity have become increasingly less viable, or even unthinkable.

The traditional parties, having lost the capacity to perform identifying representative functions (Pizzorno, 1993) in their own right, were not even able to recover their legitimacy by connecting to collective identities constituted outside of them in a public sphere that has become independent of their control (Manin, 1995). They failed to construct meaningful links with groups and social movements that articulate social interests (della Porta, 2001; Sartori, 2005). Despite the gradual erosion of electoral consensus (Bordignon, Ceccarini & Diamanti, 2018; Schadee, Segatti & Vezzoni, 2019), these parties have nevertheless managed to maintain their position of power through typical tools of the cartelisation scenario for a few decades, which has (temporarily) guaranteed the stability of the party system, albeit at the cost of reducing popular sovereignty (Mair, 2013).

In the meanwhile, participation from below has persisted, and has developed in the wake of the rise of the "critical citizens" (Norris, 2011) and models of citizenship based on the attempt to creatively balance the pursuit of collective goals and individual self-fulfilling objectives (Bennett & Wells 2009; Micheletti & McFarland, 2012). The tendency to invest the sub-political spheres of one's existence with political meaning (Beck & Beck-Gernsheim, 2002; Stolle & Micheletti, 2013) and the tendency to claim the right and responsibility to make decisions (for example, pertaining to health care, consumption and children's education) for oneself, which were once generally delegated to institutions and social conventions, increasingly characterise political participation practices. The ambition to generate change in this way relies more on the coherence between personal choices and political ideals, or on the creation of niche environments and prefigurative domains (Yates, 2021; Monticelli, 2022), than it does on seeking links with the institutional dimension of representation.

Instead, it is participation in institutionalised forms, which is also the form that is connected directly to the circuit of democratic representation, that is experiencing a contraction, both in Italy and more generally in the context of Western Europe (Mair, 2013). In conjunction with the crisis regarding the relationships between parties and participatory networks at the grassroots level, this has led to (traditional) parties that are less legitimised and more exposed to waves of anti-political and neo-populist protests (Mudde & Kaltwasser, 2013), thus paving the way for the tumultuous success of "anti-establishment" political forces, or forces that self-define as such, in 2013 and 2018: examples are the Movimento 5 Stelle (5 Stars Movement, or 5SM) followed by the Lega (League; see Bordignon et al., 2018; Schadee et al., 2019). However, the same dynamic has led to political-institutional systems that are more self-referential, less permeable to demands from below, and less bound to voters by the duties of responsiveness and accountability, which are the two sides of responsibility. Furthermore, the prevailing response to these transformations has not been to seek ways to reinvigorate grassroots participation and encourage the accountability of elected officials to voters, but the opposite. There has been an attempt to redefine democracy towards a model that is capable of being adapted to the increasing disconnection between its popular pillar and the constitutional one, whereby the former (the government "by the people") loses ground and its retreat finds a counterbalance in the latter (the government "for the people"), thus configuring a democracy in which the *demos* is no longer at the centre (Mair, 2013).

It is in this context that the transition to post-democratic scenarios takes shape (Crouch, 2005), in which the forms and procedures that are typical of representative democracy remain unchanged while they are emptied of content due to the combined outcome of the erosion of popular sovereignty, the decline (and increasing irrelevance) of institutionalised forms of participation, and the rise of a technocratic governance style that is increasingly based on direct relationships amongst public decision makers, interest representatives and experts (Bickerton & Accetti, 2021). The displacement of prerogatives towards arenas and levels that are different from the nation-state and towards actors that are disengaged from the traditional mechanisms of democratic legitimation presents a picture in which the vacuum left by forms of participation from below is replaced by the renewed prominence of interest groups and lobbies close to corporate and financial interests, which are increasingly organised on a supranational or global level. In a context marked by unprecedented levels of concentration of wealth at the global level (Piketty, 2021), the pervasiveness of globalised capitalism, financial super-entities and "philanthrocapitalism" (Dentico, 2020; Shiva, 2022) gains the capacity to influence national agendas, as well as national and supranational public regulatory agencies, which would have been difficult to imagine until a few decades ago (Galli & Bochicchio, 2016). Moreover, this process is supported by the contextual shift from traditional governmental multilateralism (the classic form of governance of supranational bodies, in which nation-state representatives participate), to "multistakeholderism", in which private actors flank state representatives in the governance of leading supranational bodies such as the UN, the WHO or the World Bank (Matteucci & Missoni 2022, 156f.).

3. Dissent or fake news?

From 2020 to 2022, in Italy and elsewhere, many protest initiatives were linked to criticisms of the management of the pandemic. During this period, these protests were amongst the most significant examples, also in numerical terms, of participation from below, with episodes of mobilisation distributed across the Italian territory for extended periods, particularly in the summer and autumn of 2021. Such protest events were repeated on a weekly basis, leading up to the attempts, real or symbolic, to block port activities in some Italian cities between October and December 2021 (Morsello & Giardullo, 2022; della Porta & Lavizzari 2022). This continuous presence in the city squares has been accompanied by intense participatory activity online, consisting of mail bombing, the launching and support of petitions, court actions, the sharing of posts on social networks sites (SNS), and coordinated actions in virtual environments, which were facilitated (and to some extent coordinated) by the establishment of a growing number of "alternative" information sources, such as web portals, television, newspapers and radio; these messages were disseminated via Facebook groups and chats on WhatsApp, as well as extensively on Telegram (Pilati & Miconi, 2022).

Across Italian regions, formalised and non-formalised groups were established around these networks, and were linked to the proliferation of initiatives aimed at training and counter-information, often in the form of courses and workshops dedicated to the in-depth study of legal and health issues with different and opposite approaches to the mainstream (Lello et al., 2022). In addition, starting from these experiences of self-organisation from below and closely tied to the local context, educational experiments aimed at providing children and the youth with alternative educational pathways to state schooling have been established. These pathways have taken shape through outdoor education organisations, particularly the establishment of parental primary and secondary schools, which are experiencing a decidedly significant spread (Chinazzi, 2021), particularly considering that the children/youth exiting the traditional schooling system to enter home-schooling, which is often not organised at the level of individual families but at the level of networks of families, has tripled in Italy following the pandemic, increasing from 5,126 children/youth in the 2018–2019 school year to 15.361 in 2020–2021.[4]

Nonetheless, in the public debate, the experiences, demands, proposals and reasons for opposition expressed by these social groups, which have included a significant minority of the Italian population, have passed almost unremarked. Very little media attention was paid to the demonstrations, even when they managed to attract relatively significant numbers of participants, except for reserving space and attention when circumstances allowed the demonstrators to be criminalised as violent and hegemonised by extreme right-wing groups.[5] In other cases, the slant of news reports and talk shows was designed to ridicule their point of view through a caricature-like portrayal, which they claimed to contrast with the opposite narrative, which was interpreted by authoritative, communication-savvy and often outnumbered personalities. Thus, news coverage was generally driven more by the intent to arouse scandal and indignation towards the so-called "anti-vaxers" than by the goal of stimulating critical reflection with some room for in-depth analysis; also considering that "anti-vaxers" became an umbrella definition applied to an increasing number of individuals, initially those who were actually unvaccinated but later extending to anyone who contested the government's management of the pandemic.

Nor did such silence (or biased and stigmatising coverage) in the journalistic information arouse significant public indignation within the public opinion, because the common feeling was that these movements were not expressing dissent, but were merely conveying attitudes of ignorance, anti-science and selfishness. Again, the "exceptionalism" of these forms of activism justified their invisibility, and precluded the need to ask questions about who these committed protesters were and what they were asking for.

However, rather than being an exception, these dynamics resembled an acceleration of what had already been observed prior to the pandemic, particularly if we focus on the relationship between protest movements and the political system. Technocratic tendencies – the outcome of the evolutions described in the

4 See Eugenio Bruno, Boom dell'homeschooling in Italia: alunni triplicati con la pandemia (Homeschooling boom in Italy: Pupils triple with pandemic), *Il Sole24Ore*, Sept. 16, 2021, https://bit.ly/3yYE6F8 (12 February 2025).

5 See Niccolò Bertuzzi, Gli utili idioti neofascisti e il futuro delle lotte contro il "green pass" (Neofascist useful idiots and the future of struggles against the "green pass"), https://bit.ly/3WqOfE6 (12 February 2025).

previous section – which result in the concentration of power in the decision-maker/expert/representative of vested interests triad, have progressively based their legitimacy on the supposed objectivity of technical expertise and scientific evidence over the years.

As government decisions have been presented as objective because "science or experts tell us so", dissent has increasingly experienced difficulty being perceived and represented as such. In addition, technical and scientific "truth", particularly if understood in a monolithic way (Bucchi, 2010), cannot be countered with legitimately different reasons: the space for dissent has gradually evaporated, leaving room only for bad faith, ignorance and fake news.

The precursors of this way of managing dissent thus appeared much earlier than the outbreak of the Covid-19 pandemic and the related protests. This discourse applies particularly to Italy, where signs began to be noticed as early as the marginalisation of the alter-global movement in 2000–2002, which became increasingly clear as the main Centre-Left party – the PD – contributed to the naturalisation of the neoliberal narrative as the only viable option over the past two decades, thus relegating critics of the dominant development model to the realm of utopian illusions, pauperism/primitivism and cultural pessimism. By that stage, there had already been (largely successful) attempts to weaken the political and antagonistic scope of movements through their delegitimisation, which was accomplished via presenting caricatures of their exponents, the recourse to categories of morality, security and "decency" (Bukowski, 2019) and, increasingly, accusations of anti-science and ignorance. An example of this was the No-Tav, a movement that opposed the Turin-Lyon high-speed railway: it is one of the most important, long-established and representative environmentalist networks in Italy (della Porta & Piazza, 2007), whose criticisms were dismissed as being based on ignorance. Similar dynamics apply to other movements that have arisen in response to large infrastructures/events, as well as to "hysterical" feminists, supporters of "degrowth" and the spheres of agro-ecology and anti-speciesism (della Porta et al., 2019; Bertuzzi, 2018).

Thus, the prevailing portrayal of protests against pandemic policies in the public discourse, while forming a continuum with pre-existing dynamics, also represents a moment of significant acceleration and dramatisation. The causes can be traced to the increased centrality acquired by science (and medicine, which is considered to be even more objective and less debatable than is science in a broad sense) as a justification for policy making, together with the contextual changes that have caused science to become one of the privileged arenas for lobbying penetration strategies.

4. Between science and lobbying, between participation and participatory washing

Recent technocratic and biopolitical tendencies, to which the COVID-19 health crisis has imparted an acceleration that is particularly evident in the Italian case, have relied on the supposed objectivity of appealing to the evidence or data, which would in itself be sufficient to legitimise government decisions by exauthorising the role of public debate.

However, in addition to the difficulties implicit in considering scientific evidence as an objective source for policy making (Wynne, 2014), one must consider the risks inherent in the scientisation of policy (Pielke, 2005); that is, the attempt by politics to nullify conflict by resorting to science as a synonym for unquestionable truths, thus concealing those decisions that are laden with value and political choices behind a veil of supposed objectivity (Hobson-West 2003; Saltelli & Sarevitz, 2022).

However, the objectivity of scientific knowledge must also be problematised in light of the fact that it is precisely on the spheres of the production and governance of scientific knowledge that the most innovative and pervasive strategies of influence insist, particularly those of "regulatory capture"[6] carried out by the corporate sectors. In turn, these are closely implicated in the semantic overturns with which we began.

Since the 1990s, organisations linked to the chemical, fossil fuel, agricultural products and pharmaceutical industries have invested in the "merchants of doubt" strategy: they have produced scientific evidence to challenge and question the methods and results of academic and independent research demonstrating the health and environmental hazards of substances such as tobacco, pesticides and GMOs (Oreskes & Conway, 2010). To achieve this, these industries have exploited the information asymmetries between regulatory bodies and lobbying organisations, so that the former are often forced to rely on evidence provided by the same manufacturing companies under their control, as they lack the necessary funds to develop research directly (Saltelli et al., 2022). The notion of "sound science" can be traced to this period, and was paradoxically coined by tobacco industrialists to contrast with alleged "junk science", a term that was used to describe research warning of the dangers of passive smoking (Foucart, Horel & Laurens, 2020).

6 Dal Bò (2006, 203) defined regulatory capture as "the process through which special interests influence public intervention in any of its forms, in areas as diverse as fiscal policies, choices concerning foreign policy or monetary policy, or legislation concerning research and development".

Faced by the controversy triggered by the exposure of the conflicts of interest of the researchers involved, the corporate sector has refined and broadened the scope of its actions, to the extent that the merchants of doubt strategy is now considered to be only the first step on an "epistemic ladder" that lobbies have climbed in the most recent period (Saltelli et al., 2022). In the second step (the institutional strategy), industrial interests pointed to blur the distinction between the controllers and the controlled, and aimed to counter their image as special-interest bearers to the point of presenting themselves as defenders of the public interest within science; thus, they have attempted to colonise the domains in which the governance of science and the relationships between it and public regulation are defined. Finally, through the political strategy (the third step), they aimed to change the broader context and worldviews via the endorsement of principles such as the innovation principle, which challenges the precautionary principle, with the aim of imposing a neoliberal, market-centric gospel in which even public regulation is presented as undesirable and, therefore, liable to be depowered.

Such strategies found a powerful complement in a range of activities targeted at colonising the public sphere through the "cultural capture"[7] of ordinary citizens (Foucart, Horel & Laurens, 2020). In order to silence any criticism, and to ensure that corporate interests were widely relaunched from below, the strategy evolved by leveraging the opportunities offered by the emergence of SNSs and the professionalisation of digital influence. Specialised agencies serving the corporate sector have thus favoured the packaging of "scientific evidence" from industry-sponsored research, or at least selected on the basis of results, which are nevertheless disseminated without an explicit indication of the sources and funding channels, and are presented as a block of unchallenged knowledge from a monolithic "scientific community" in formats that are ready for dissemination through SNSs or to the press. Following the insight (developed in the marketing field) that the most effective strategy to sell a product in the current context, is to entrust its promotion not to celebrities but to ordinary citizens, who are perceived as more trustworthy because they are deemed to be disinterested, the privileged targets of lobbying penetration strategies have become (quasi)ordinary "science lovers". They are people who enjoy some credit due to their online profiles without being scientists or specialists in the field, and are eager to promote the role of science in public debate and to defend it from the attacks that, according to this narrative, would be perpetrated by groups driven by ignorance, irrational and anti-scientific fears, or corporate interests. This is what constitutes

7 This expression describes the process whereby the target of capture actions comes to see the world in the same way as the lobbyists do, not because of corrupt actions but because he or she has been convinced (Dal Bò, 2006, 220).

"astroturfing" (literally "fake grass", Walker, 2014), which is a strategy whereby elite interests are promoted through a network of micro-influencers that includes animators of science popularisation blogs, fact-checkers and volunteer debunkers who are enlisted as "guardians of reason" without their knowledge (Foucart, Horel & Laurens, 2020), to the point of giving the illusion that the same questions and demands stem from grassroots activism. One can speak of participatory washing in this regard.

It is in this way that it has become possible for the most polluting and health-threatening industries on the planet to pursue their interests by appealing to the value of science and the rationalist ideas that used to be part of the Left's heritage, and are now being used in a real semantic overturn as a result of "language capture". Thus, they can silence and stigmatise social movements, journalists and activists who attempt to denounce the risks and harm associated with their products, resulting in them being accused of "fear marketing", hysteria and spreading fake news (Foucart, Horel & Laurens, 2020; Dentico, 2020).

Similar dynamics occur in "non-Western" contexts. In some countries of the Global South, agricultural programmes such as AGRA,[8] which was launched by global philanthrocapitalism, advocate, in the name of science, the need to increase productivity (to defeat hunger) through glyphosates, monocultures, genetic engineering, technologies and market ideology, without any consideration of the damage that industrial agriculture has already done to biodiversity and soil fertility. As is evident in the *Monsanto Papers*, the need to pursue this path is defended through smear campaigns against those who critically study its effects. At the same time, those "resistant peasants" (Scott, 1986) denounce the "genetically modified colonialism" of an approach that stigmatises local knowledge and any form of thought based on the recognition of the earth as a living being, as a tradition to be eradicated in the name of progress and scientific thought. This is despite the fact that, in the 13 countries covered by the AGRA programme, hunger has increased by 30% instead of decreasing (Dentico, 2020).

In the health field, the gradual marginalisation of the WHO's role, combined with actions aimed at its capture by philanthropic foundations and the complex network of public-private partnerships linked to them, has resulted in the WHO's objectives tending to increasingly coincide with those of the foundations themselves (Missoni et al., 2019; Dentico & Missoni, 2021). Some African and Asian countries, in which health systems have been dismantled as a result of impositions placed by the World Bank as a condition for access to loans, have become the purview of philanthropic programmes that establish health reform strategies that are mainly aimed at promoting the private sector and generating new markets. Thus, public health strategies tend to be reduced to the "elegant

8 https://agra.org/ (12 February 2025).

tool" of vaccines (Dentico, 2020, 150ff.), while no attention is paid to the fundamental determinants of health such as access to clean water, sewage systems and adequate nutrition, or to the restructuring of local health systems, not even for the distribution of vaccines, which instead emblematically travels, as per the "Last Mile" project, on Coca-Cola's distribution networks (ibid., 154f.). The semantic impoverishment of the concept of public health, which tends to be condensed into that of immunisation, thus overlaps with philanthropy as a continuation by other means of the hegemony exercised by the corporate sector.

The influence of philanthrocapitalism, as the result of its enormous financial resources, even pollutes the processes of scientific knowledge production in the field of health; an example is the goal of malaria eradication launched by the Bill and Melinda Gates Foundation. According to the former WHO's chief of infectious diseases, Kochi Arata, such dynamics threaten the necessary pluralism of approaches and opinions and impair the quality of peer review mechanisms, as well as denoting a scientific imperialism of initiatives conceived according to a Western cosmology and implemented in disregard of local knowledge and epistemologies (Dentico, 2020; Kaul et al., 2022).

In the name of science and sustainable development, in the agricultural field, as well as in the field of health care, industrial sectors use philanthrocapitalism to target sick or starving sectors of the planet driven by the intent to create new markets and financial products in a powerful re-enactment of Western colonialism that was effectively reconstructed in its scope and consequences by Vandana Shiva (2020; 2022).

5. Implications for the public sphere and participation

The aforementioned changes regarding parties, social movements and interest/pressure groups, as well as their mutual relationships, are at the origin of the processes of "language capture" that use concepts and symbols of the Left to promote green/ethics washing, to which participatory washing has been added more recently.

In this second part of the chapter, we focus on some of the implications of these processes for the functioning of the public sphere, as well as for the conditions and opportunities for mobilisation, and then see how the application of this perspective can be useful for interpreting mobilisations around pandemic policies.

Based on the arguments thus far, traditional Left-wing struggles such as defending the value of science and rationalism, public health, environmental protection and "sustainability", have become battlegrounds for multiple political subjectivities, thus generating a confusing and difficult-to-read situation that results in the pollution and hijacking of the public sphere.

Instead of the traditional opposition between the reasons for environmental protection (or public health) versus those of the market and the private sector, or between the defence of science versus religious or ethno-identitarian instances, a new scenario has tended to emerge. Movements and collective actors attempting to articulate an emancipatory and anti-capitalist discourse about these issues find themselves being increasingly pitted against political forces that continue to refer to the broad field of the Left and progressive politics and to claim the same keywords, albeit transformed into empty shells designed to legitimise the interests of extractive capitalism (Klein, 2015). An example is ecological movements that find themselves opposed to the idea of "ecological transition" based on nuclear power, food bio-fortification, genetic engineering and green capitalism (Leonardi, 2017; Keucheyan, 2019).

The conflict thus shifts between the world that recognises itself in the signifiers of progressive politics by interpreting them (in practice but not explicitly) according to a neoliberal framework, and those circles that attempt to elaborate an emancipatory and anti-capitalist criticism; the latter are often discredited and delegitimised precisely because, by virtue of their antagonistic positions with regard to the progressive (mainstream) field, they are assimilated in a simplistic and one-sided way to the Right, or even to the extreme Right, as well as to ignorance and conspiracy theories (Bertuzzi et al., 2022; Lello & Bertuzzi, 2025). Overall, in these cases, citizens and activists experience loneliness because they cannot find support from the civil society organisations with which they have often shared long paths of political activism. These organisations are bound and trapped in that "language capture", as well as in the situation of confusion and disorientation that it fuels. Thus, the possibility of politically countering the interests of neoliberal governance is further hampered in a context in which battles are waged under false flags and elitist interests are disguised as demands from below; thus, those who seek to provide a genuinely emancipatory critique find themselves robbed of their own words. For example, consider the criticisms of agribusiness, which have been downgraded as being attributable to an "organic lobby" or, conversely, ecological practices such as those of biodynamic agriculture, which have been opposed and labelled as "anti-scientific" (Breda, 2017).

The same loneliness has been experienced by many of the citizens who have taken to the physical and virtual public squares to criticise some of the policies adopted to manage the pandemic crisis. These policies have been cloaked in solidarity and progressive rhetoric, but they appear to be consistent with the objectives of restructuring Western capitalism in an authoritarian and oligarchic way (Green & Fazi, 2023). These citizens have expressed demands for more attention to be paid to the pluralism of the scientific debate surrounding different health policies and their consequences – as well as about the dangers of increasing digitalisation and surveillance technologies – but experienced the barrier of a caricatural representation of monolithic science, yet one made more indisputable through science lobbying and astroturf dynamics (Gandini & Miconi, 2022).

6. Mobilisations against pandemic policies

If it is in the "language capture" that the reasons for the hegemony of a simplistic and stigmatising view of pandemic management critics must be sought, it is the unravelling of these dynamics that makes it possible to trace the boundaries of a different interpretation of these protests, one that links them to the on-going redefinition of the lines of political conflict and contextual processes of re-politicisation.

Mobilisations related to vaccine hesitancy and opposition to pandemic policies are heterogeneous in terms of identities and political orientations, and are not exempt from dynamics of extremism and conspiracy-like degeneration. In this regard, while it is important to avoid the *tout court* assimilation of protests as a conspiracy, it is equally important to adopt a conscious and critical approach to the classist view attached to a particular use of the category of "conspiracy" (Lagalisse, 2019), as well as a perspective that is capable of recognising the role of power relations in determining the likelihood that certain theories are labelled as such (Pelkmans & Machold, 2011; Lello & Saltelli, 2022).

We draw on qualitative research based on 67 semi-structured interviews that were conducted between 2020 and 2021 with vaccine-hesitant Italian people (more details and a broader discussion of the methods and results are available in Lello et al., 2022), as well as on earlier qualitative-quantitative research concerning participants in protests against the extension and tightening of the paediatric vaccination requirements that were introduced by Law No. 119/2017, better known as the Lorenzin reform (Lello, 2020).

In the subjective motives and representations of these segments of the population, the empirical analysis highlights the relevance of several of the themes mentioned here, thus allowing one to identify attempts, however embryonic, to thematise emancipatory claims pertaining to crucial issues that have received little or no attention in the political debate. The emancipatory stances, which generally receive little consideration in the stereotypical representation of these protests, are linked to the not insignificant weight of biographies stemming from Leftist, environmentalist and critical consumption circles (Lello, 2020; Lello & Bertuzzi, 2025).

A widely felt theme is the criticism of developments that are perceived as degenerative and reductionist in health care, but which also affect medicine in general. In the pre-pandemic mobilisations that were mainly related to paediatric vaccines, the negative consequences of the corporatisation and privatisation of health care, as well as the weight and intrusiveness of pharmaceutical lobbies, had already been thematised, together with other aspects that were related more to the paradigm and practices of biochemical medicine (Cavicchi, 2022). These criticisms included the hyper-sectorisation that loses sight of the relationships amongst the parts, the deterministic and materialistic conceptions of the human being, the protocol-based and depersonalising approach, the focus on the symptoms while neglecting the causes, and the marginalisation of primary prevention. A significant proportion of our interviewees grafted a more conscious scepticism of Western biochemical medicine onto these almost unanimously shared critiques, which was sustained by adherence to competing epistemologies or epistemic communities (Navin, 2016; Sobo, 2016; Attwell et al., 2018) based on different conceptions of the body and health. In this case, health is interpreted according to a holistic view of the human being, not only with regard to the physiological components, but also in terms of the emotional, psychological, social and spiritual dimensions, and is actively pursued via an emphasis on aspects related to lifestyle, nutrition and the different components of primary prevention. In many cases, although not always or necessarily, these views were linked to the use of complementary and alternative medicines (CAM; see Attwell et al., 2018).

More recent protests against pandemic policies have included a broader range of issues than strictly medical-health ones, but these continue to be relevant, as evidenced by the significant continuity between these mobilisations and the traditional vaccine hesitancy circles (Troiano & Nardi, 2021). Due to the pandemic, the increasing politicisation of the issue has reverberated in generally more radical, conscious and far-reaching stances, thus revealing the consequences of pathways of re-politicisation that are altering subjective perceptions and narratives (Lello et al., 2022). Thus, widespread criticism of the undue pervasiveness of capitalism in health care, as well as in medicine itself has emerged, together with denunciations of authoritarian evolutions involving health care institutions. These denunciations concern the repression of debate and informational pluralism, the divestment of channels of confrontation amongst different positions, as well as the denigrating campaigns against CAMs, and extend to the disbarment of physicians who expressed perplexity or caution regarding vaccination policies rather than about vaccines, as summarised in the interview excerpt below:

> There are, for example, doctors from Ippocrate.org who are not against vaccines, they would like another type of vaccine that offers guarantees, and yet no one is listened to, not only that, they are threatened. I'll tell you more, another doctor […] was banned because he said that there is no active pharmacovigilance, not even that there isn't: that it's done wrong, however, it's not that the institutions respond by showing that "look you were wrong, active pharmacovigilance is there", no, since you said that active pharmacovigilance isn't there I'm going to ban you, I'm going to suspend you, I'm going to punish you, and it has to be clear that those who speak are not trustworthy. […] What have I noticed over the years? That I used to be able to say that I had been a victim of the vaccine and I had people around me, where I went I went, who had no problem telling me "but you know me too and me too", and even doctors would respond to me […] and there were even webpages that explained it, now what happened? The webpages that used to talk about the consequences of polio vaccination […] are gone, gone […] and I didn't even think about doing prints years ago, I couldn't think at that time that these webpages could disappear, […] and the thing that makes me cringe is […] the inability of younger doctors to realise that the vaccine can have consequences. (int., male, 60 year-old)

A strongly shared and related concern regards the power of lobbies, as well as global philanthrocapitalism and the influence on supranational and national bodies, which is perceived as excessive and lacking adequate counterweights, thus resulting in denunciations of the decline of democracy and the shrinking of popular sovereignty.

The influence of organised interests is also at the centre of the thematisation of science, highlighting an orientation that deviates considerably from the stereotypical image of the "no-vaxxer": widespread belief in scientific research and methods *per se* has emerged (Lello, 2020), while doubts and perplexities pertain to the conditioning by lobbies and power structures in the areas of the construction and dissemination of scientific knowledge. Hence, as early as 2017, a demand for participation in the elaboration of the research agenda took shape in order to invest in the analysis of the subjective variables associated with the likelihood of developing adverse reactions to vaccines, or in active drug-vigilance programmes. More recently, due to the pandemic, criticisms have tended to focus on the imbalance of power in favour of multinational pharmaceutical companies, and thus on the lack of transparency and capacity on the part of regulatory bodies in imposing contractual conditions that would strike a balance between profits and the interest of the population in terms of ensuring adequate safety standards.

Opposition to 5G technology, but more generally to the digitisation of society and to an uncritically techno-optimistic perspective, also stems from a broader scepticism about the purposes of a technological "advancement" that is suspected of leading to social scenarios that will be characterised by further accelerations of the rhythms of life, production and consumption, as well as by new possibilities for surveillance and control to the detriment of the autonomy of individuals and communities (Lello et al., 2022). What appears to be in question is the socio-technical imaginary (Jasanoff & Kim, 2015) that defines technological progress as a value to be sustained in itself, thus hinting at the emergence of a demand for the opening of a debate about the underlying social purposes, benefits, spillovers and costs of these choices.

7. Conclusions

The analysis presented in the previous sections clarifies the desirability of (re)setting aside functionalist keys and related perspectives focused on the psychological or even pathological aspects of participants in protests against pandemic policies. Far from representing an exception on the road to the emergence of the critical citizen – as well as on the one leading to the emergence of the "demanding" patient in the medical field (Stacey et al., 2009; Cavicchi, 2010) – these protests represent a possible outcome of these same processes.

Besides, the denial of these protests as expressions of legitimate political demands is not really an exception: we are experiencing an acceleration of dynamics that were already noted in past decades, in which the growing disconnect between government and participation was accompanied by the increasing assimilation of dissent into the categories of fake news and ignorance.

It is in this context that a semantic reversal of signifiers traditionally belonging to the Left occurred, which later received significant impetus from the growing centrality of science in decision-making combined with a renewed aggressiveness of scientific lobbying.

A first consequence of this language capture concerns the increased difficulty of politically challenging the decisions of neoliberal elites. That is, it has become more arduous to articulate a genuinely emancipatory criticism due to the delegitimisation of protest, the semantic confusion that is being created in the public sphere and the opening up of fracture lines within areas and networks that were previously united by mutual recognition in the (broad) horizons of the Left.

Moreover, relevant context changes, that induce and nurture forms of repoliticisation and mobilisation, are also being created. For this reason, it would arguably be more fruitful to turn to theories that link the emergence of social protests, as well as their paths of consolidation and radicalisation, to changes in the political opportunities structure instead of recovering functionalist perspectives (della Porta & Diani, 2015).

The impact of those context changes on the landscape and conditions for mobilisation can be highlighted in at least two ways. On the one hand, those same changes in neoliberal governance prompt counter-responses in the form of critical reactions and requests for thematisation, as effectively evidenced by the centrality, in the visions of pandemic protesters, of the denunciation of the weight of lobbying, philanthrocapitalism, and the entanglement of scientific, medical and capitalist interests.

On the other hand, a change in context that is as relevant as it has hitherto been little considered concerns the medical-scientific sphere. In the Italian mobilisations against paediatric vaccination in 2017, well-founded reasons for overcoming the mainstream interpretation of these protests as being driven by anti-science and ignorance, could be identified in the recognition of the elements of rationality and in the questions of an insuppressibly political nature that were linked to the existence of alternative expert systems and, more generally, to specific tensions and inadequacies in the biochemical medicine paradigm in relation to the specifics of the contemporary social context (Lello 2020; Cavicchi, 2022). While protests during the COVID-19 pandemic embraced a broader audience than the traditional vaccine hesitants, including dubious positions concerning only specific vaccines – or even only concerning sanction and control policies, such as the so-called Green Pass – the elements of criticism involving medical-health issues remain central.

As a first point, the politicisation of healthcare choices, which began with the extension of (paediatric) vaccine requirements in 2017 and accelerated in accordance with the COVID-19 pandemic, has removed the question of personal adherence to epistemologies of care and health from the realm of individual choice. As a result, the context of the "healthcare bricolage" (Colombo & Rebughini, 2006) in which citizens, even without being fully aware of the epistemological gaps that differentiate approaches and practices of care, switch from one to the other based on predominantly empirical considerations supported by directly experienced efficacy, has become less and less viable.

Moreover, in order to understand the contextual change that has taken place from a broader perspective, it is necessary to start from the evolutions, summarily mentioned here, that have led the WHO towards the gradual adoption of a reductionist approach to the issue of health, and to increasingly distance itself from its own definition of health in 1977, as well as from the Alma Ata declaration in the following year, in which a vision centred on equity, community participation and prevention was proposed in relation to the whole social and economic development of the community (Alma Ata, 1978; see also Matteucci & Missoni, 2022). A significant juncture, in order to contextualise the progressive impoverishment of the concept of "health" and its parallel move closer to that of "immunisation", must therefore be identified in the changes in the sphere of global health governance, which have led to a progressive coincidence between the goals of the WHO and those of the corporate sector, organised in the complex network of public-private partnerships and programmes revolving around philanthrocapitalism (Dentico & Missoni, 2021).

These global processes reverberated and found a specific declination according to the particular dynamics of the Italian context, which was selected as a global vaccine policy leader in the agreement signed by the Global Health Security Agenda (GHSA) in 2014. In Italy, political and communicative choices have tended towards the adoption of authoritarian models, perhaps in the hope of hastily "blocking" growing dissent and tensions amongst epistemological approaches. The adoption of communicative registers that authoritatively represent science as dogma (as exemplified by the well-known virologist and science populariser Roberto Burioni), the smear campaigns against CAMs, the blocking of experiments involving the integration and complementarity between biochemical medicine and CAMs within public health, all the way to the banning of physicians expressing not entirely orthodox positions concerning vaccines, represent elements that are likely to profoundly change the context, acting as stimuli for mobilisation (and radicalisation to some extent), particularly for those segments of society that are not completely comfortable with the biomedical paradigm and that practice different epistemologies of health in their daily lives.

This type of response on the part of health institutions signals an attempt to react to biochemical medicine's crisis of credibility and legitimacy by blocking the channels of dialogue with the different views, and opposing anything that does not fit into an even more restrictive and orthodox declination of the same biochemical medical paradigm to which they refer. It is in this way that not only adherence to alternative expert systems, but also dissent with the encroachment of neoliberalism in the field of health, have been labelled *tout court* as ignorance to be eradicated and repressed. The result has been an authoritarianism devoid of authority, which increasingly allows one to observe the extreme fragility of the feet of clay on which it rests.

Subsequent political and communicative choices have fuelled paths of radicalisation, and have led to significant minorities of the population no longer being able to recognise themselves in health (or political) institutions, or in the mainstream media environment, thus pushing them toward the search for alternative information channels. This is to say that, by continuing to blame the "conspiracy theorists", one feeds conspiracy theories or, more realistically, one feeds an alternative information network that, being unable to engage in dialogue and confront itself with more "official" points of view due to the stigma and exclusion to which it is subjected, is exposed to paths of radicalisation. Apart from eroding the legitimacy and credibility of institutions, this results in the fragmentation of the public sphere that undermines the conditions for the existence of the evidence of discussion that Manin (1995) identified as being amongst the fundamental principles of representative government.

In conclusion, if it is necessary to question the categories that are used to think about these protests, one starting point may be to recognise an outcome of justification of existing power relations and dominant interests in the recovery of functionalist approaches; this outcome is consistent with the history of structural-functionalism, as Wright Mills (1962) critically pointed out. In this case, "language capture" appears to have taken the form of using Leftist ideas such as solidarity, public health, and a generally hoped-for "return of the state" after decades of market primacy, to justify and support pandemic policies. However, these policies should more plausibly be interpreted as the outcome of decades-long processes of capture by organised private interests, which increasingly seek to use public (both state and supranational) institutions and agencies to pursue their goals of increased profits and creation of new markets (Green & Fazi, 2023). The result is a situation of great confusion and pollution within the public sphere, in which it becomes as difficult as it is important to articulate a coherent position of support for public intervention that is capable of representing the interests of the community while simultaneously limiting and countering the intrusiveness that structures that can be traced to global financial capitalism exert, even within the state apparatuses themselves.

Works cited

Agnoletto, V. & Guadagnucci L. (2010). *L'eclissi della democrazia.* Milano: Feltrinelli.

Alma Ata (1978). *Primary Health Care.* Report of the International Conference on Primary Health Care. USSR, Alma Ata.

Attwell, K. & Smith, D.T. (2017). Parenting as politics: social identity theory and vaccine hesitant communities. *International Journal of Health Governance*, 22, 3, 183–98.

Attwell, K., Ward, P.R., Meyer, S.B., Rokkase, P.J. & Leask, J. (2018). Do-it-yourself: Vaccine rejection and complementary and alternative medicine (CAM). *Social Science and Medicine*, 196, 106–14.

Beck, U. & Beck Gersheim, E. (2001). *Individualization: Institutionalized Individualism and its Social and Political Consequences.* London, New York: Sage.

Bennett, L. & Wells, C. (2009). Young Citizens and Civic Learning: Two Paradigms of Citizenship in the Digital Age. *Citizenship Studies*, 13, 2, 105–120. doi: 10.1080/13621020902731116.

Bertuzzi, N. (2018). *I movimenti animalisti in Italia. Strategie, politiche e pratiche di attivismo.* Milan: Meltemi.

Bertuzzi, N., Lagalisse, E., Lello, E., Gobo, G. & Sena, B. (2022). Politics During and After Covid-19: Science, Health and Social Protest. *Partecipazione & Conflitto*, 15, 3, 507–529. doi:10.1285/i20356609v15i3p507.

Bickerton, C.J. & Accetti Invernizzi, C.I. (2021). *Technopopulism: The new logic of democratic politics.* Oxford: Oxford University Press.

Bordignon, F., Ceccarini, L. & Diamanti, I. (2018). *Le divergenze parallele. L'Italia: dal voto liquido al voto devoto.* Roma-Bari: Laterza.

Breda, N. (2017). The plant in between: Analogism and entanglement in an Italian community of anthroposophists, *Anuac*, 5, 2, 131–157. doi:org/10.7340/anuac2239-625X-2530.

Bucchi, M. (2010). *Scientisti e antiscientisti. Perché scienza e società non si capiscono.* Bologna: Il Mulino.

Bukowski, W. (2019). *La buona educazione degli oppressi.* Roma: Alegre.

Caruso, L., Giorgi, A., Mattoni, A. & Piazza G. (2010). *Alla Ricerca Dell'Onda. I nuovi conflitti nell'istruzione superiore.* Milano: FrancoAngeli.

Cavicchi, I. (2010). *Medicina e sanità snodi cruciali.* Bari: Dedalo.

Cavicchi, I. (2022). *La scienza impareggiabile.* Roma: Castelvecchi.

Chinazzi, A. (2021). *Home Education: Reshaping Teachers and Parents' Responsibilities in the Era of Intensive Parenting.* The European Conference on Education 2021 Official Conference Proceedings.

Colombo, E. & Rebughini, P. (2006). *La medicina contesa. Cure non convenzionali e pluralismo medico.* Roma: Carocci.

Coniglione, F. (ed.) (2010). *Through the Mirrors of Science. New Challenges for Knowledge-based Societies.* Heusenstamm: Ontos Verlag.

Crouch, C. (2005). *Post-democrazia.* Roma-Bari: Laterza.

Dal Bó, E. (2006). Regulatory capture: A review. *Oxford Review of Economic Policy*, 22, 2, 203–225. doi: org/10.1093/oxrep/grj013.

Della Porta, D. (2001). *I partiti politici.* Bologna: Il Mulino.

Della Porta, D., & Piazza, G. (2007). Local contention, global framing: The protest campaigns against the TAV in Val di Susa and the bridge on the Messina Straits. *Environmental Politics*, 16, 5, 864–882. doi:10.1080/09644010701634257.

Della Porta, D. & Diani, M. (2015). *The Oxford Handbook of Social Movements.* Oxford: Oxford University Press.

Della Porta, D., Piazza, G., Bertuzzi, N. & Sorci, G. (2019). LULUs Movements in Multilevel Struggles: A Comparison of Four Movements in Italy. *Rivista Italiana di Politiche Pubbliche*, 3, 477–513. doi:10.1483/95213).

Della Porta, D. & Lavizzari, A. (2022) The protests against anti-contagion measures and vaccination in Covid19 times: Waves of contention in Italy 2020–2021. *Partecipazione & Conflitto* 15, 3 bis, 720–740. doi: 10.1285/i20356609v15i3p720.

Della Porta, D., Bertuzzi, N., Chironi, D., Milan, C., Portos, M., & Zamponi, L. (2022) *Resisting the Backlash: Street Protest in Italy.* Routledge.

Dentico, N. (2020) *Ricchi e buoni? Le trame oscure del filantrocapitalismo.* Verona: EMI.

Dentico, N. & Missoni, E. (2021). *Geopolitica della salute: Covid-19, OMS e la sfida pandemica.* Soveria Mannelli: Rubbettino.

Fava, T. (2013). *Il Partito Democratico visto dal basso.* Roma: Aracne.

Floridia, A. (2019). *Un partito sbagliato. Democrazia e organizzazione nel Partito Democratico.* Roma: Castelvecchi.

Foucart, S., Horel, S.& Laurens, S. (2020). *Les gardiens de la raison: enquête sur la désinformation scientifique.* Paris: La Découverte.

Hobson-West, P. (2003) Understanding vaccination resistance: moving beyond risk. *Health, Risk and Society*, 5, 3, 273–83. doi.org/10.1080/13698570310001606978.

Galli, G. & Bochicchio, F. (2016). *Scacco alla superclass. La nuova oligarchia che governa il mondo e i metodi per limitarne lo strapotere.* Milano-Udine: Mimesis.

Green, T. & Fazi, T. (2023). *The Covid Consensus: The Global Assault on Democracy and the Poor. A Critique from the Left.* Hurst.

Inglehart, R. (1977). *The silent revolution: changing values and political styles among western publics.* Princeton, NY: Princeton University Press.

Jasanoff, S. & Kim, S.-H. (2015). *Dreamscapes of Modernity. Sociotechnical Imaginaries and the Fabrication of Power.* Chicago: University of Chicago Press.

Katz, R.S. & Mair, P. (1995). Changing Models of Party Organization and Party Democracy. The Emergence of the Cartel Party. *Party Politics*, 1, 1, 5. doi: 10.1177/13540688950 01001001.

Katz, R.S. & Mair, P. (2009). The Cartel Party Thesis: A Restatement. *Perspectives on Politics*, 7, 753. doi: 10.1017/S1537592709991782.

Kaul, S., Akbulut, B., Demaria, F. & Gerber, J. F. (2022). Alternatives to sustainable development: what can we learn from the pluriverse in practice? *Sustainability Science*, 17, 4, 1149–1158. doi.org/10.1007/s11625-022-01210-2.

Keucheyan, R. (2019). *La natura è un campo di battaglia.* Verona: Ombre corte.

Kitschelt, H. & MacGann, A.J. (1995) The radical right in Western Europe: a comparative analysis. The University of Michigan Press, Ann Arbor, MI. doi: 10.3998/mpub.14501.

Klein, N. (2015). *This changes everything: Capitalism vs. the climate.* New York: Simon and Schuster.

Lagalisse, E. (2019). *Occult Features of Anarchism: With Attention to the Conspiracy of Kings and the Conspiracy of the Peoples.* PM Press.

Latouche, S. (2011). *Décoloniser l'imaginaire: La pensée créative contre l'économie de l'absurde.* Parangon.

Le Bon, G. (1895). *Psychologie des foules*, Alcan; trans. It. *Psicologia delle folle.* Longanesi, 1980.

Lello, E. (2020). Populismo anti-scientifico o nodi irrisolti della biomedicina? Prospettive a confronto intorno al movimento free vax. *Rassegna Italiana di Sociologia*, 61, 3, 479–508.

Lello, E. & Bertuzzi, N. (eds.) (2022). *Dissenso informato. Pandemia: il dibattito mancato e le alternative possibili.* Roma: Castelvecchi.

Lello, E. & Saltelli, A. (2022). Lobbismo scientifico e dirottamento dello spazio pubblico. In E. Lello, & N. Bertuzzi. (eds.), cit., (pp. 187–203).

Lello, E., Bertuzzi, N., Pedroni, M. & Raffini, L. (2022). Vaccine hesitancy and refusal during the Covid-19 pandemic in Italy: Individualistic claims or repoliticisation? *Partecipazione & Conflitto*, 15, 3, 672–696. doi: 10.1285/i20356609v15i3p672.

Lello, E., & Bertuzzi, N. (2025). From Big Farms to Big Pharma? Problematizing science-related populism. *Public Understanding of Science.* https://doi.org/10.1177/096366252 51316727 (05 March 2025).

Leonardi, E. (2017). *Lavoro, natura, valore: André Gorz tra marxismo e decrescita.* Napoli-Salerno: Orthotes.

Mair, P. (2013). *Ruling the void: The hollowing of Western democracy.* Verso books.

Manin, B. (1995). *Principes du gouvernement répresentatif.* Paris: Flammarion.

Matteucci N. & Missoni E. (2022). *Strategie di cattura e governance multistakeholder: il caso dell'OMS.* In E. Lello & N. Bertuzzi (eds.), cit., (pp. 151–166).
Micheletti, M. & MacFarland, A.S. (2012). *Creative Participation. Responsibility-taking in the Political World.* New York-London: Routledge.
Missoni, E., Pacileo, G., & Tediosi, F. (2019). *Global health governance and policy: an introduction.* London: Routledge.
Monticelli, L. (ed.) (2022). *The Future Is Now: An Introduction to Prefigurative Politics: The Future Is Now.* Policy Press.
Morsello, B. & Giardullo, P. (2022). Free choice in the making: Vaccine-related activism as an alternative form of citizenship during the Covid-19 pandemic. *Partecipazione e conflitto*, 15, 3 bis. doi: 10.1285/i20356609v15i3p697.
Mudde, C. & Kaltwasser, C.R. (2013). Populism. In M. Freeden, L.T. Sargent & M. Stears (eds.), *The Oxford Handbook of Political Ideologies* (pp. 493–512). Oxford: Oxford University Press.
Navin, M. (2016). *Values and Vaccine Refusal: Hard Questions in Ethics, Epistemology and Health Care.* New York: Routledge.
Norris, P. (2011). *Democratic Deficit. Critical Citizens Revisited.* Cambridge: Cambridge University Press.
Oreskes, N. & Conway, E.M. (2010). *Merchants of doubt. How a handful of scientists obscured the truth on issues from tobacco smoke to global warming.* Bloomsbury.
Pelkmans, M. & Machold, R. (2011). Conspiracy theories and their truth trajectories. *Focaal*, 59, 66–80. doi:10.3167/fcl.2011.590105.
Pielke, R.A.J. (2005). *Scienza e politica.* Roma-Bari: Laterza.
Piketty, T. (2021). *Une brève histoire de l'égalité.* Paris: Éditions du Seuil.
Pilati, F. & Miconi, A. (2022). The "Green Pass" Controversy in the Italian Twittersphere: a Digital Methods Mapping. *Partecipazione e Conflitto* 15, 3, 549–566. doi: 10.1285/i20356609v15i3p549.
Pizzorno, A. (1993). *Le radici della politica assoluta e altri saggi.* Milano: Feltrinelli.
Saltelli, A., Dankel, J.D., Di Fiore, M., Holland, N. & Pigeon, M. (2022). Science, the endless frontier of regulatory capture. *Futures*, 135, 102860. doi.org/10.1016/j.futures.2021.102860.
Saltelli, A. & Sarewitz D. (2022). Reformation in the Church of Science. *The New Atlantis*, 68, 56–64. https://www.thenewatlantis.com/publications/reformation-in-the-church-of-science (22 March 2024).
Sartori, G. (2005). Party Types, Organisation and Function. *West European Politics*, 28, 1, 5–32. doi.org/10.1080/0140238042000334268.
Schadee, H., Segatti, P. & Vezzoni, C. (2019). *L'apocalisse della democrazia italiana. Alle origini di due terremoti elettorali.* Bologna Il: Mulino.
Scott, J. (1986). Everyday forms of peasant resistance, *The Journal of Peasant Studies*, 13, 2, 5–35. doi.org/10.1080/03066158608438289.
Shir-Raz, Y., Elisha, E., Martin, B., Ronel, N. & Guetzkow, J. (2022). Censorship and Suppression of Covid-19 Heterodoxy: Tactics and Counter-Tactics. *Minerva*, 1–27. doi: 10.1007/s11024-022-09479-4.
Shiva, V. (2020). *Filantrocapitalismo come ricolonizzazione.* Introduction in N. Dentico, cit.

Shiva, V. (2022). *Philanthrocapitalism and the Erosion of Democracy.* Santa Fe: Synergetic Press.

Simis, M.J., Madden, H., Cacciatore, M.A., & Yeo, S.K. (2016). The lure of rationality: Why does the deficit model persist in science communication? *Public understanding of science*, 25, 4, 400–414. doi: 10.1177/0963662516629749.

Sobo, E.J. (2016). Theorizing (vaccine) refusal: Through the looking glass. *Cultural Anthropology*, 31, 3, 342–350. doi.org/10.14506/ca31.3.04.

Stacey, C.L., Henderson, S., MacArthur, K.R., & Dohan, D. (2009). Demanding patient or demanding encounter?: A case study of a cancer clinic. *Social science & medicine*, 69, 5, 729–737. doi: 10.1016/j.socscimed.2009.06.032.

Stolle, D. & Micheletti, M. (2013). *Political Consumerism. Global Responsibility in Action.* New York: Cambridge University Press.

Troiano, G. & Nardi, A. (2021). Vaccine hesitancy in the era of COVID-19. *Public Health*, 194, 245–251. doi: 10.1016/j.puhe.2021.02.025.

Walker, E.T. (2014). *Grassroots for hire: Public affairs consultants in American democracy.* Cambridge: Cambridge University Press.

Wynne, B. (2014). Further Disorientation in the Hall of Mirrors. *Public Understanding of Science*, 23, 1, 60–70. doi.org/10.1177/0963662513505397.

Wright Mills, C. (1962). *L'immaginazione sociologica.* Milano: Il Saggiatore.

Yates, L. (2021). Prefigurative politics and social movement strategy: The roles of prefiguration in the reproduction, mobilisation and coordination of movements. *Political Studies*, 69, 4, 1033–1052. doi.org/10.1177/0032321720936046.

Local Perspectives

Łukasz Kumięga

Right-Wing Extremism and Vaccine Opponents / Corona Deniers in Germany: An Outline of Postlinguistics

Abstract
The following article addresses the question of the possibility of establishing a postlinguistic perspective within critical and empirical research, especially of public discourses. The approach draws on reflections on Critical Linguistics and Critical Discourse Studies starting with current social challenges, and is illustrated with an analysis of an interview, which reveals the microdiscursive, interdiscursive and macrodiscursive effects of the entanglement of discourse on right-wing extremism with the discourse of vaccine opponents and Corona deniers in Germany, interpreting it as one of many examples that visualize and legitimize postlinguistic intervention.

Keywords: Critical Discourse Analysis, Critical Linguistics, language, power, criticism, right-wing extremism, anti-vaccination discourse, Postlinguistics.

1. Introduction

The COVID-19 pandemic has become a "discursive event"[1] (Jäger, 2012, 76) due to its status as a subject of public debate. In order to establish a "discursive event", a certain field of "sayability" is necessary, that is to say there exists the possibility "to speak about" the "event", transforming it into a communicative phenomenon. In the case of the COVID-19 pandemic, this field of "sayability" appeared almost automatically due to its global and far-reaching relevance, whereby (and this is of particular interest to discourse studies) further discourse progression uncovered some exemplifications with regard to its possible (and impossible) shifts in the field of sayability. It is precisely at this point that the question of the scope of a linguistically-founded and socially relevant critique arises again (see the article by Warnke in this volume and Czachur 2020). It is in

Łukasz Kumięga, University of Gdansk, ORCID: 0000-0002-8034-3593.

1 All of the German-language quotations in this article have been translated into English by the author of the article.

this context that this article invites us to refresh the academic debate on the limitations and potential of linguistics when dealing with "explosive topics" (Jäger, 2012, 157–162), which is shown here using examples and data related to discourse on the COVID-19 pandemic in Germany. This will also include an attempt to present an outline of postlinguistics.

2. Sources of postlinguistics

Postlinguistics, understood primarily as a linguistically and socially sensitive view of how reality is constructed, is based in particular on approaches drawn from critical linguistics and critical discourse studies. This conceptual way partly shows a certain development within the approach to language, also partly within linguistics.

The critical way of linguistics can be traced back, in particular, to the approaches of critical linguistics (cf. for example Fowler et al., 1979; or Kress & Hodge, 1979). If one locates this in time, it must be noted that it sought to establish itself in the context of a certain dominance of structuralism and the slow establishment of the communicative-pragmatic turn. A certain linguistic basis of this approach is provided by reflections on language and its functions. Here, language is understood as an activity which paved the way for the establishment of the systemic functional perspective within linguistics. The following three meta-functions of language have been differentiated (cf. Halliday & Hasan, 1989): the ideational function, which includes the articulation of views on the world, references to knowledge complexes and belief systems; the interpersonal function, which addresses the implication of subject positions, social and situational roles and identities as well as the construction of relationships between the participants; and, finally, the textual function, which concerns the provision of elements and structures for the location of utterances (sentences) in an ensemble (a text, an interaction). In this way, language is clearly included in a social context, which for critical linguists means an invitation to further specification. On the one hand, a strong linguistic foundation of this perspective is emphasised (at the same time linked to a broad contextualisation), by assuming that the linguistic structure is analysed in detail in the light of the social and historical situation of a text. On the other hand, cognitive-axiological aspects are also emphasised, since for critical linguistics the patterns of meaning and the values encoded in language constitute a fundamental subject area. Finally, it defines the crucial function of critical linguistics, which is to shed light on discourses that those who take them for granted lose sight of, and to regard their reconstruction and, above all, their deconstruction as an empirical task (Fowler et al., 1979, 17).

On this basis, various approaches to "critical discourse studies" have been established internationally, and within this framework, and with particular reference to the underlying theory formation[2]. A distinction is made between six research programmes[3], each of which has a slightly different theoretical emphasis (Wodak, 2017). In order to grasp the relevant moment of a specific accentuation of this perspective, it is necessary to expand on the somewhat reductionist approach from the point of view of the current state of research in linguistics, which, however, historically reveals a certain paradigm shift within linguistics, especially empirical linguistics, and which Wodak (2017, 54) refers to as "dispositive analysis". Thus, Jäger and Zimmermann (2010) distinguish between linguistics (understood as language analysis) and discourse analysis (understood as propositional analysis[4]), i.e. they refer to the potential of linguistic elements (words, sentences, texts) for empirically conditioned continuation (via context or, for example, collective symbols) and, as a result, to reconstruct the structure of the semantic depth of the discourse. For example, at demonstrations by so-called "corona deniers" (in German: "Coronaleugner"), the following sentence is often heard: "Stop the vaccination genocide"[5]. From a discourse-critical point of view, this is above all a decontextualisation and recontextualisation of the primary meaning of vaccination, which is associated with immunisation and protection. Instead, it accuses them of killing and even genocide. The mechanisms of the health care system, previously regarded as protective mechanisms, thus become an occasion for a linguistically based, politically motivated and socially consequential instrumentalisation. This makes it clear that discourse analysis (in its critical variant) seeks to contribute to the reconstruction of social processes that are constructed through language (cf. Duszak, House & Kumięga, 2010).

Furthermore, the linguistic construction of society is integrated into processes of inclusion and exclusion (linked, for example, to the reproduction of various hierarchical and institutionally anchored orders), thereby expressing its strategic

2 Wodak (2017, 54) attempts to identify the following sources of theory in this regard: M. Foucault, critical theory, K. Marx, S. Moscovici, symbolic internationalism, M.A.K. Halliday.

3 The Discourse-Historical Approach (R. Wodak, M. Reisigl, M. Rheindorf, M. Krzyżanowski), Corpus Linguistics Approach (G. Mautner, P. Baker), Social Actor Approach (T. Van Leeuwen), Dispositive Analysis (S. Jäger, F. Maier), Socio-Cognitive Approach (T.A. Van Dijk), and the Dialectical-Relational Approach (N. Fairclough), cf. Wodak, 2017, 54.

4 Jäger and Zimmermann illustrate this with the example of the media discourse on the GDR (demonstrations in Berlin against the SED leadership on 17 June 1953) and explain it with the title of the article from "Die Zeit" (16 February 2006): "Steine gegen rote Panzer" ("Stones against red tanks") as follows: "The phrase 'stones against red tanks' (context, collective symbol) refers to the statement 'the weak against the strong' and thus makes visible the potential of the so-called propositional analysis" (Jäger & Zimmermann, 2010, 16).

5 https://kurier.at/chronik/oesterreich/verfassungsschutz-warnt-coronaleugner-haben-kranke haeuser-im-visier/401812234 (24 December 2024).

side. At this point, we come to the transition to the discursive moment of deconstruction alluded to above. Deconstruction needs a basis for the process of deconstruction. The first open question at this point is: does science have sufficient tools to enable a deconstructivist perspective on social discourses?

3. Postlinguistics between Philosophy of Science and Criticism in Linguistics

It is no coincidence that this question is posed here, since, among other things, critical discourse analysis, in particular, has had to go through a somewhat difficult path in order to establish itself as a critical research perspective in the discursive and non-discursive (power-related) field of science (especially linguistics). This was and still is partly related to the somewhat outdated dichotomies regarding the scientific approach, such as Description vs. Critique, Description vs. Prescription, or Objectivity vs. Subjectivity, which are readily invoked in the theory of science and are formulated according to disciplinary orders. At this point, in the context of the postlinguistics discussed in this article, reference is made to Popper (1994/1996), who formulated stimulating considerations of a scientific-theoretical nature: "There is no such thing as a purely observational [empirical] science; there are only sciences in which we theorize (more or less consciously and critically). This also applies to the social sciences" (Popper, 1994/1996, 78). Here two aspects become explicit and implicit: the scope of a critical attitude, which (as I understand it) is to be scientifically determined and substantiated, and the transferability of these reflections to all scientific disciplines, i. e. to linguistics. Furthermore, Popper (1994/1996) suggests that the objective and value-free scientist is not the ideal scientist because s/he lacks "passion". Even if the category of "passion" is not to be regarded here as a scientific category, it is primarily a metaphorical way of making clear that objectivity and value-neutrality are themselves values. And since value-neutrality is itself a value, the demand for unconditional value-neutrality in Popper's argument is "paradoxical". This makes it relatively clear that it is difficult for science to understand itself as an "entity" independent of the discursive order and society, one capable of producing value-free discourses. To put it bluntly, and in the sense of the postlinguistics postulated here, I see science as a place of close interplay between scientific analyses and deconstructions of the socially relevant fields closely associated with it (see also Spitzmüller & Warnke, 2011, 13–63).

Building on these initial considerations, the next step is to refer to the stereotypical oppositions of description and critique elaborated by Reisigl and Warnke (2013, 18), which point to the linguistic and discursive mechanisms of social (including scientific) reality. In my opinion, the term "stereotypical oppositions" (because of their questioning) opens up the way for a scientifically sound examination of this problem, because it corresponds in part to the aspect formulated by Popper on the scope of the critical stance. The oppositions mentioned are explained as follows: the so-called "description" is associated with superficial structures, with the visible and perceptible, with neutrality and being value-free, as well as with objectivity, something uninteresting, non-normative, affirmative, uncritical, ahistorical, realistic and descriptive. In line with and in contrast to this, a so-called "critique" is seen as an attitude associated with backgrounds/deep structures, the invisible/hidden, judgments and subjectivity, as well as with a commitment to interests, prescriptiveness, reflexivity, historical orientation, utopia and interpretation, and explication/argumentation.

As the first assessment of the partial aspects introduced so far, it can be said that the postlinguistics discussed here, especially in the context of linguistic research and its scientific and social positioning, is part of the following series of meta-aspects, which can be formulated as questions: How does criticism manifest itself in language? Which social and scientific objects correspond to criticism? How is the scope of criticism to be understood in this way? To what extent can criticism be scientifically substantiated?

Some answers to these questions can be found in the context of linguistic approaches to discourse semantics and discourse linguistics. This can clearly be interpreted as a relevant opening in the field of linguistic thinking (or, to put it provocatively: it should be appreciated). Felder (2009) in the context of the discussion about the critical in linguistics (using language criticism as an example) distinguishes between language criticism as a contribution to language awareness and language criticism as social criticism. The first perspective is concerned with the judgment of words, phrases, texts and discourses, taking into account the context of language use and criteria related to appropriateness and success. The second perspective focuses on the attitudes and identities of a cultural community that are communicated through language. It can be said to be about reconstructing the "self-image" of a linguistic and cultural community (including from a comparative perspective). Dreesen (2013) models the critical in linguistics in an even more specific way by distinguishing the following four areas: "non-prescriptive linguistic criticism", by which he means pointing out the alternatives to language use; "critical through description", which means raising awareness of political attitudes and discursive processes by, for example, scientific analysis that arrives at a different idea of knowledge about immigration than the widespread one; "critical through contrastive linguistics", i.e. the comparison of two different discourses, and finally, "overarching critique", understood as a critique of existing specialized academic knowledge (e.g. of the German Language Association). As a very relevant step with regard to the critical attitude within linguistic research, which is scientifically founded and regarded as a stimulus for postlinguistics, two proposals in particular can be identified here: 1) the discourse-critical potential for pointing out alternatives in the linguistic construction of social reality, and 2) the discourse-critical potential for constructing alternative scientific interpretations of social reality that can deconstruct a certain dominance of the interpretations presented so far.

4. Why postlinguistics?

The logic of the conceptual inscription of postlinguistics in the scientific field is based on the semantic-logical mechanisms of postmodernism, poststructuralism and postfeminism. If we look at the prefix "post", it is used to denote (in formations with adjectives – more rarely with nouns or verbs) something that takes place later in time (https://www.duden.de/rechtschreibung/post_#google_vignette, 28 December 2024). This temporal dimension is central here, and in the context of the development of linguistic thought, because it indicates that postperspectives are not primarily concerned with questioning what is "before" but rather with specifying or re-accentuating what is "before" in a contemporary way. In addition, and in relation to one of the possible objects of linguistics, i.e. the aspect of the linguistic construction of social reality, the temporal dimension is relevant insofar as it corresponds to the temporal development of the social system. The term "post-truth times", which has been somewhat overused in recent years, should be considered here, since it paradoxically plays a role (through the use of the same prefix) in the context of the term postlinguistics and thus covers the area that should be the actual subject of the postlinguistic perspective. Post-truth times relate to so-called "alternative facts" that stand in contrast to so-called "real facts". Here too, paradoxically, a contrast is created that is, at first sight, counter-discursive. What is real in discourse and what is alternative? After all, discourse-critical approaches to research are also about reconstructing alternatives.

This may sound logical, but it is more complex than that. In reality, as constructed here with postlinguistics, it is a matter of uncovering mechanisms that make it possible to reinforce what is constructed as "real" or to exclude what is constructed as "alternative", or to reinforce what is constructed as "alternative" and ultimately to exclude what is constructed as "real". Going one step further, the question arises as to whether there should be an axiological component in constructions of particularly socially relevant relations along the four relations defined above, on which postlinguistics should draw.

Let us take as an example the particularly sensitive field of medicine which is the subject of this volume. The COVID-19 pandemic has been constructed in various discourses of populist, radical and right-wing extremist movements as following an "alternative" logic, for example by referring to it as a "corona hoax" (https://www.tagesschau.de/faktenfinder/corona-schwindel-101.html, 28 December 2024)[6] in relation to certain conspiracy theories (with all the discursive and non-discursive effects associated with this). Does the task of linguistics, and thus of postlinguistics, end with the mere identification of the linguistic constructions of the COVID-19 pandemic? Is it enough to describe the discursive mechanisms of these constructions in the form of peer-reviewed articles in linguistic journals? Or do we perhaps need a strong post-linguistic voice in society that, on the one hand, reconstructs the "alternative" constructions and, on the other hand, "passionately" (to return to Popper) takes a position on them, in order, for example, to discursively counteract the possibility of endangering the health system in the context of the COVID-19 pandemic? It is only here – I hope – that it becomes relatively clear which component has been missing in linguistic research to date.

In summary, I propose to reinterpret so-called "actionism" (in German "Aktionismus", cf. Kumięga, 2023, 44–51), understood in a discourse-linguistic context as a reproach to critical research (cf. e.g. Warnke, 2007), and to bring more to the fore its partial meaning of "endeavoring to change people's consciousness or existing conditions through [provocative, revolutionary, artistic] actions" (https://www.duden.de/rechtschreibung/Aktionismus, 30 December 2024). "Actionism" may seem too hasty, but it has the social task of responding to certain states of emergency (in the Foucauldian sense). Moreover, the basic component of "actionism" is "action", i.e. an activity or otherwise "concerted action" (especially in politics[7]; joint action achieved via the agreement of all partners; coined in 1967 by Karl Schiller, https://www.duden.de/rechtschreibung/Aktion, 30 December 2024). The negatively connoted scientific "actionism" can therefore also mean that linguistics (here construed as postlinguistics) has to understand that in certain emergencies it has to take action by using its specialised and expert knowledge in a socially relevant way and by contributing to the deconstruction of alternative facts.

Many aspects of the discursive approach are based on such a perspective:

- Russell's (1911) proposed categorisation of types of knowledge into knowledge from experience, knowledge from cognition, and knowledge from (linguistic) description, which is integrated into discourse linguistics research with the argument that it is primarily knowledge from linguistic description that

6 An open question in this context is whether tagesschau.de is acting unscientifically from the point of view of the post-linguistics postulated in the article.

7 Of course, this "definition" can be criticised for having political overtones. The politicisation of various social subsystems is a problem that is becoming increasingly visible in post-factual times and should not be lost or forgotten in the eyes of science (including linguistics).

constitutes the constructions of modern societies (Spitzmüller & Warnke, 2011, 13–63);
- the first point corresponds to the theoretical framework of discourse-based approaches, which is linked to constructivism: "the linguistic constitution of reality is understood as a practice of making statements in oral or written form, in which statements format phenomena as reality through specific purposes of action" (Spitzmüller & Warnke, 2011, 45);
- the dialectical relationship between language and society is emphasised: "on the one hand, social processes manifest themselves in discourse, on the other hand, discourse simultaneously represents these processes" (Wodak, 2017, 55);
- the critical stance is primarily based on Kant's concept of critique (critique as a reflexive examination of the conditions of the possibility of knowledge (see e. g. Kant, 2020) and its Foucauldian power-analytical specification: critique as "the art of not being governed quite so much" (Foucault, 2007 [1978], 45). In relation to the post-linguistic perspective, it is about not being governed by forces that demand a deconstruction of the social order;
- in discourse-critical approaches, the content of critique is defined monodiscursively, for example as "the attempts of the right to control people's thinking" (Beaugrande, 2008, 108) or as "explosive topics" (Jäger, 1999). Postlinguistics promotes the multidiscursive perspective in this respect, for example by making the exclusionary processes of neoliberal discourses the subject of empirical approaches[8];
- science is seen as a discursive field of interest-bound positions. These interests do not necessarily have to be negative, but can also be seen as a basis for counteracting the massive spread of post-factual content (Nowicka-Franczak & Kumięga, 2020);
- critical scholarship, including critical discourse analysis, will only remain socially relevant if it has something new to say about new developments. It must therefore look beyond its own horizons and, above all, take up other approaches (from other sciences and cultural traditions) in an interdisciplinary way, critically reflect on them, take them into account and, if necessary, integrate them (Wodak et al., 2010, 561–562).

The aspects addressed here range from the epistemological foundations to constructivism and the associated power mechanisms to the concrete content

8 Other important aspects of this perspective include issues such as the pedagogisation(s) of society, the normalisation(s) of populism, the normalisation(s) of exclusion, and the economisation(s) of science.

and positioning of the discourse-critical approach and thus justify the possibility of opening up linguistics to the post-linguistic perspective.

5. Right-wing extremism and COVID-19 pandemic discourse

The empirical framework of this article is based on the observation of a specific relationship between right-wing extremism and discourse on the COVID-19 pandemic. Before examining this relationship in more detail and empirically, it is important to identify which elements of right-wing extremist discourse form the basis for further reflection. Within the discourse on right-wing extremism (using the example of state institutions such as the Federal Office for the Protection of the Constitution and academic institutions), three types of discourse can be distinguished: normative discourse, moderate discourse and critical discourse (cf. Kumięga, 2013, 72–76). These are conceptually different and construct the relationship to left-wing extremism in a differentiated way, but are united in defining the basic elements of right-wing extremist discourse. These include ethnocentrism and racism, the subordination of the individual, the glorification of the nation, anti-pluralism and homogeneity. Looking at right-wing extremist discourse in more detail and on the basis of an empirical study (see Kumięga, 2013), the following aspects can be distinguished as core elements of right-wing extremist identity discourse:

- ideological identity concepts containing many heterogeneous and, at first sight, mutually exclusive elements: National Socialism/nostalgia for the Third Reich, anti-Semitism/pacifism, a pro-Palestinian position;
- opponent-oriented identity concepts (anti-Americanism, an anti-systemic attitude towards the Federal Republic of Germany and its "supporters", anti-Israelism);
- parliament-oriented identity concepts (references to the NPD);
- action-oriented identity concepts (calls for direct action, space-oriented activities, strengthening of the sense of community);
- experience-oriented identity concepts (implicit calls to violence, implicit signalling of the willingness to use violence);
- subcultural identity concepts (e.g. references to the skinhead subculture);
- pop-cultural identity concepts (references to pop-cultural discourses);
- modernization-oriented identity concepts (borrowings from democratic discourses, from discourses of political opponents, integration of mainstream concepts);
- individuality-oriented identity concepts (pluralisation).

6. Empirical illustration: on the qualitative potential of the postlinguistic perspective

If right-wing extremism is linked to the antivax discourse – as it is in the interview analyzed – then the question arises as to which elements of the right-wing extremist discourse make this link possible. The reconstruction of this connection and the postlinguistic perspective on it is one of the aims of the empirical part of this article. This problem is illustrated by an interview with Dr Alexander Yendell[9] from the University of Leipzig, which is available on the YouTube channel[10] of Deutsche Welle[11] (published on 9 December 2021, 188,618 views[12]). In the case of such an institution-related (university) constellation, which is publicly and mass (media) mediated, we are dealing with interdiscourse[13], which is assigned the task of making subject-specific content[14] accessible to the general public, in particular through linguistic and discursive mechanisms (of "translation", also understood as simplification[15]). One of the most important tasks of a postlin-

9 https://fgz-risc.de/das-forschungsinstitut/personen/details/alexander-yendell (30 December 2024). The self-presentation of the interviewer available here shows his rather macrostructural view of right-wing extremism (underpinned by individual conditions that are methodologically validated on the basis of standardised survey data) (e.g. via the references to democracy research) and his expertise in the field of diverse (qualitative and quantitative) social research: "Destruction of democratic structures") and his expertise in the field of diverse (qualitative and quantitative) social research.

10 Also on Facebook: /deutschewellenews; Twitter:/dwnews and Instagram: /dwnews (29 December 2024).

11 https://www.youtube.com/watch?v=3FJOhWqI0JM&t=210s (29 December 2024).

12 The number of views is actually irrelevant in the context of this article. Rather, the aim is to capture the publicly visible logics of such discourses, which signals the qualitative orientation of the analysis to come.

13 This de-differentiating, partially reintegrating tendency of knowledge production, which runs counter to the tendency of knowledge specialisation, leads to the paradoxical constitution of separate discourses whose specialty is, so to speak, non-specialty and which can be called interdiscourses (Link, 1988, 284–307). Well-known examples are popular religion, popular philosophy, popular history, pedagogy, journalism, conversation (now talk shows), art and literature, and later popular science, media politics and media entertainment. Obviously, modern differentiated cultures of expertise cannot be confined exclusively to specific fields of knowledge, but in order to reproduce them, they also require reintegrating fields of knowledge as a kind of correlate or compensation, which mediate between the specialties and "build bridges" (Link, 2013, 11).

14 These are briefly introduced in the interview by discussing the specifics of scientific work, referring to aspects such as: quantitative research, population surveys, representativeness, political attitudes, sampling, testing scientific theories and criticism within the scientific field.

15 When discussing the scientific basis of his explanations, Dr Yendell emphasizes: "It's not something we make up at our desks. The specificity of interdiscourse lies therefore also in the use of colloquial forms", https://www.youtube.com/watch?v=3FJOhWqI0JM&t=210s (29 December 2024).

guistic perspective is to critically analyse the logic of such an interdiscourse and to question its social function, especially since it creates various discontinuities and contradictions with regard to the field "discussed" (in the case of the present interview, the links between the far-right scene and the so-called "Corona deniers"), which require a postlinguistic intervention.

Let us begin the analysis with a thematic (discourse strand related) reconstruction of the structure of the interview, which is superfluous insofar as it is given on the YouTube channel when the respective interview sections are determined (in the form of questions by the DW journalist) and largely corresponds to the content of this interview. The elements of this structure are

- Introduction;
- Aren't all vaccine opponents extremists?
- Is this coming from Corona deniers?
- How do you research?
- Why do people believe in conspiracy theories?
- How does the scene radicalise?
- Has the network become more professional in the era of the coronavirus?
- How important is the anti-corona movement?
- To what extent could Corona deniers again become the starting point for further radicalisation?
- What strategies do politicians need to develop?
- Which components of a worldview are indicative of a radical right-wing worldview?
- Why do these attitudes seem to find such fertile ground in East Germany?
- Are you, as a political scientist, threatened?[16]

If one tries to systematise this structure even further, the following picture emerges: right-wing extremism and its links to Corona deniers/vaccine opponents, the specifics of Corona deniers/vaccine opponents, conspiracy theories, political strategies against Corona deniers/vaccine opponents, scientific-research and scientific-individual aspects as well as the East German context.

The core of the detailed analysis of the interview consists of the following categories, which I believe follow a pattern that is particularly relevant to knowledge, which seeks to connect the micro-level with the macro-level via the interlevel and then the:

- micro-level: nominalisations: how are social actors – individuals and groups – named or linguistically constructed? (Reisigl, 2007). This is a rather underestimated category, because, although it is relatively "easy" to reconstruct from an analytical point of view, it provides fundamental insights because it im-

16 https://www.youtube.com/watch?v=3FJOhWqI0JM&t=210s (29 December 2024).

plicitly visualises semantic relations in the discursive field, which form an important basis for the contouring of social reality;
- inter-level: discourse entanglements and their power effects: Discourse strands never appear individually. Rather, they are intertwined, influence and support each other and thus produce specific discursive effects. It is therefore important for the analysis not only to consider discourse fragments on the topic under analysis, but also to pay attention to entanglements with other topics (Jäger, 1999, 99). This is the second category (from the perspective of broad discourse research) of fundamental analytical categories, because it is context-related (e.g. public debate) and includes the other scientifically founded categories such as intertextuality and interdiscursivity (in contrast to the above-mentioned category of interdiscourse) and, in particular, from the perspective of discourse-critical research, empirically addresses the moment of linguistic and discursive power formation;
- macro-level: the category of the "dispositive of the political" (Kumięga, 2013) is used here, which opens up a macro-perspective. The macro-level is important because it makes it possible to see language and discourse as elements of broader social and political mechanisms. This is also the great advantage of analyses of this kind, because they are always embedded in the macro-social processes that they seek to explain interpretatively.

In what follows, all the aspects presented will be explained and justified in terms of their potential for the post-linguistic perspective.

At the micro-level mentioned above, we are interested in the way in which the political scene "to the right of the Union" (Hirsch, 1989) is constructed linguistically. In this respect, we encounter a rather broad semantic disorder that can be linguistically categorised as denotational competition. This mechanism consists in attributing different labels to a certain phenomenon or to a certain social or political group. In the interview analysed, Dr Alexander Yendell refers arbitrarily to "right-wing extremists", "right-wingers", "populists" or "radicals".[17] The DW journalist constructs this field by using terms such as "right-wing terrorists"[18] or "right-wing radicals".[19] In general, it should be noted that in more everyday texts, a labelling competition is used to demonstrate an author's broad semantic competence. In the analysed interdiscourse, this is problematic because, despite the specificity of the interdiscursive relations, conceptual consistency is not only desirable but even necessary, especially since the scientific conceptualisation (especially within political science and extremism research) of

17 https://www.youtube.com/watch?v=3FJOhWqI0JM&t=210s (29 December 2024).
18 The Federal Minister of the Interior is quoted in this context.
19 https://www.youtube.com/watch?v=3FJOhWqI0JM&t=210s (29 December 2024).

right-wing extremists, right-wing populists, right-wing radicals or further right-wing extremists has completely different semantic and conceptual, but also political, characteristics. This semantic disorder and arbitrariness may have a strategic function, which could be to create different discursive effects in order to discredit the scene to the right of the Union through semantic attribution, but instead it leads to semantic chaos and thus to a blurring of the field under discussion and its diverse conceptual reception.

The interview announces a focus on right-wing extremism ("How right-wing is the scene of corona deniers and 'lateral thinkers' [in German Querdenker]?"[20]), instead, competing and semantically different terms are used to construct this field linguistically. And it is precisely here that a postlinguistic voice is needed, one that is sensitive to language, understands the consequences of the linguistic construction of reality, and draws journalism's attention to the need for conceptual sensitivity.

Let us take one step further and look at the construction of interdiscursivity in the analysed interview. The title of the interview refers to these constructions in that it promises to answer the question of the extent to which the scene of corona deniers and "lateral thinkers" is right-wing extremist. From an analytical point of view, this is an attempt to link right-wing extremist discourse with the discourse of corona deniers and lateral thinkers, and to show their specific nature. This complex relationship is explained on several levels. First, at the level of the search for the connection between right-wing extremist discourse and the discourse of the Corona deniers and lateral thinkers. This means that the characteristics of right-wing extremist discourse must first be made visible, and they include according to Dr Yendell "the concept of inequality", "the trivialisation of Nazism", "anti-Semitism", "social Darwinism", "xenophobia" and "racism"[21]. However, these elements of this discourse cannot be explicitly linked to the discourse of Corona deniers and lateral thinkers. The element that links the two is seen primarily as the division of reality into "good" and "evil", which can be largely linked to the logic of conspiracy theories (see the contributions by Czyżewski and Niehr in this volume), which are defined according to Dr Yendell as "thought structures" whose main function is to "reinterpret reality"[22]: i. e. both

20 https://www.youtube.com/watch?v=3FJOhWqI0JM&t=210s (29 December 2024).

21 https://www.youtube.com/watch?v=3FJOhWqI0JM&t=210s (29 December 2024). With regard to the above-mentioned characteristics of the right-wing extremist discourse presented in Kumięga (2013), a rather reductionist perspective can be seen here, which interprets this discourse only in relation to the attitudes of the right-wing extremist actors reproduced in it and ignores its action-oriented dimension, which is able to show many other elements of the potential connection of the right-wing extremist discourse with the discourse of the anti-vaccinationists and corona deniers, for example through the "common" recourse to the form of action of a demonstration.

22 https://www.youtube.com/watch?v=3FJOhWqI0JM&t=210s (29 December 2024).

discourses can be linked via the reproduction of conspiracy theory discourse elements. The connection thus constructed is, so to speak, scientifically limited by the following statement: "of course, not all anti-vaccination activists are right-wing extremists, but there is a correlation, a connection between anti-vaccination and right-wing extremism" (Dr Yendell in the interview under analysis). This correlation is further elaborated on by addressing the following aspects in a very disorganised manner:

- instrumentalisation of anti-vaccination discourse in the context of right-wing extremist discourse (especially in its party-related variant);
- interdiscursive reinforcement of the intended correlation by referring to scientific studies that reveal the voting behavior of anti-vaccination activists, i.e. their tendency to vote for right-wing extremist parties;
- the sources of this correlation, i.e. the question as to what extent this correlation is quasi-automatically produced by the radial and extreme positions in society or whether these positions are new (i.e. as a result of the pandemic).

From the perspective of discourse analysis, the interweaving of both discourses (the right-wing extremist discourse and the discourse of corona deniers and anti-vaccination activists) leads to the construction of a category of "right-wing radical anti-vaccination activists"[23] (Dr Yendell), which can be seen as a product of the constructions mentioned in the interview. This right-wing radicalisation is also linked to violent protests and calls for murder (e.g. via posts on Telegram).

Looking at this mechanism from the perspective of discourse analysis, we are dealing here with the simple invocation of alarmist discourse, which according to Klarner & Kohlstruck (2006, 33) has the following function and thus discursive consequences in the context of discourse on right-wing extremism: "A semantic standardisation of the heterogeneous field of right-wing extremism into a closed threat figure, as is typical of public discourse, makes it difficult to gain insight into (…) the peculiarities of the various phenomena, their respective specific dynamics of emergence and the appropriate ways of dealing with them". Since right-wing extremism represents a threat to democracy from a scientific and political point of view, its interdiscursive connection with the discourse of corona deniers and lateral thinkers is quasi-logically given, because the second type of discourse mentioned in this constellation clearly inscribes itself in the need to legitimise and consolidate the security dispositive (constructed in the analysed interviews as "internal security"), which is quasi-automatically given in the case of right-wing extremism. In this respect, the mechanism reconstructed here

23 In relation to the micro-level aspects mentioned above, the use of the term "right-wing radical" can be explained here as a result of the conceptual confusion of the interview analysed.

represents a very simple way of dealing with the discourse of corona deniers and lateral thinkers. Instead of dealing with its content postlinguistically, a familiar and apparently effective pattern is used to create alarming discursive effects.

On the macro level announced above, we can speak here of the reproduction of the "dispositif of the political" (Kumięga, 2013). All the elements of this dispositive serve to defend and consolidate the status quo of the current micro-political orders, and – what is particularly relevant from the perspective of Foucault's dispositive-analytical view of the logic behind the constructions of social reality – this takes place within the framework of a specific interplay of a media, political and social setting of the elements of the dispositive, which consists in the fact that they complement and support one another. An important question in the context of this article, which must also be asked in relation to current developments in the political field, is: are these mechanisms still a suitable strategy for influencing public debates? (cf. Kumięga & Nowicka-Franczak, 2023).

7. Conclusion

The analysis carried out has made it clear that a post-linguistic voice has much to say and to achieve in the public debate. This achievement consists in particular in:
- cultivating a language-sensitive view of the conceptual construction of reality by not losing sight of conceptual and scientifically based orders and continuities;
- cultivating a content-oriented engagement with socially and politically relevant discourses in order to reveal their specificity to the recipients of the interdiscourse, to offer an off-pattern examination of social discourses that does not take the easy way out by falling back on old and no longer effective discursive (primarily media and micro-political) orders;
- in order to become a macro-politically relevant voice by discursively strengthening content-related and partially redefined orders of liberal democracy.

In this respect, this paper invites all socially sensitive linguists to become a strong macro-societal voice in the sense of postlinguistics.

Works cited

Beaugrande, R. de (2008). Krytyczna analiza dyskursu a znaczenie "demokracji" w wielkim korpusie. In A. Duszak & N. Fairclough (eds.), *Krytyczna analiza dyskursu: Interdyscyplinarne podejście do komunikacji społecznej* (pp. 103–120). Kraków: Universitas.

Czachur, W. (2020). *Lingwistyka dyskursu jako integrujący program badawczy.* Wrocław: Oficyna Wydawnicza ATUT.

Czyżewski, M. (2005). *Öffentliche Kommunikation und Rechtsextremismus.* Łodź: Wydawnictwo Uniwersytetu Łódzkiego.

Dreesen, P. (2013). Kritik als Erkenntnismodus, Praxis und Untersuchungsgegenstand in der Diskurslinguistik. In U.H. Meinhof, M. Reisigl & I. Warnke (eds.), *Diskurslinguistik im Spannungsfeld von Deskription und Kritik* (pp. 169–201). Berlin: Akademie Verlag.

Duszak, A., House, J., & Kumięga, Ł. (eds.) (2010). *Globalization, Discourse, Media: In a Critical Perspective.* Warszawa: Wydawnictwa Uniwersytetu Warszawskiego.

Felder, E. (ed.) (2006). *Semantische Kämpfe. Macht und Sprache in den Wissenschaften.* Berlin, New York: Walter de Gruyter.

Foucault M. 1997 [1978]. What is Critique? In S. Lotringer & L. Hochroth (eds.), *The Politics of Truth.* New York: Semiotext(e).

Fowler, R., Hodge, B., Kress, G., & Trew, T. (1979). *Language and control.* London, Boston: Routledge & Kegan Paul.

Halliday, M.A.K., & Hasan, R. (1989). *Language, context, and text: aspects of language in a social-semiotic perspective.* Oxford: Oxford University Press.

Hirsch, K. (1989). *Rechts von der Union. Personen, Organisationen, Parteien seit 1945. Ein Lexikon.* München: Knesebeck & Schuler.

Jäger, S. (1999). *Kritische Diskursanalyse. Eine Einführung.* Münster: Unrast.

Jäger, S. & Zimmermann, J. (eds.) (2010). *Lexikon der Kritischen Diskursanalyse: Eine Werkzeugkiste.* Münster: Unrast.

Kant, I. (2020). The Critique of Practical Reason. Frankfurt am Main: Outlook Verlag.

Klarner, A., & Kohlstruck, M. (eds.) (2006). Moderner Rechtsextremismus in Deutschland. Bonn: Bundeszentrale für Politische Bildung.

Kress, G. & Hodge, R. (1979). *Language as ideology.* London, Boston: Routledge & Kegan Paul.

Kumięga, Ł. (2023). Zur diskurskritischen Konstruktion des Begriffs des Themas. In J. Engelken, M. Glund, J. Hensellek, L. Herford, S. Langrock, S. Poghosyan, S.S. Schmalwieser, & I.H. Warnke (eds.), *Was ist eigentlich ein Thema? Sieben linguistische Perspektiven* (pp. 44–51). U Bremen Research Alliance. https://doi.org/10.26092/elib/2312 (20 May 2022).

Kumięga, Ł., & Nowicka-Franczak, M. (2023). Weighing discourse in a single-case study. An attempt at an appraisal. In Ł. Kumięga & M. Nowicka-Franczak (eds.), *Analysing discourse, analysing Poland: the case of a political interview* (pp. 269–274). Göttingen: Vandenhoeck & Ruprecht Verlag.

Kumięga, Ł. (2013). *Rechtsextremistischer Straßendiskurs in Deutschland.* Frankfurt am Main: Peter Lang.

Link, J. (2013). Diskurs, Interdiskurs, Kollektivsymbolik. Am Beispiel der aktuellen Krise der Normalität. *Zeitschrift für Diskursforschung,* 1/2013, 7–23.

Link, J. (1988). Literaturanalyse als Interdiskursanalyse. Am Beispiel des Ursprungs literarischer Symbolik in der Kollektivsymbolik. In G. Fohrmann H. & Müller (eds.), *Diskurstheorien und Literaturwissenschaft* (pp. 284–307). Frankfurt am Main: Suhrkamp Fohrmann/Müller.

Nowicka-Franczak, M. & Kumięga, Ł. (2020). Od redaktorów: analiza dyskursu a prawda o dyskursie. *Przegląd Socjologii Jakościowej, 16*, 6–17. https://doi.org/10.18778/1733-8069.16.4.01 (10 June 2022).

Reisigl, M. (2007). Projektbericht: Der Wiener Ansatz der Kritischen Diskursanalyse. *Forum Qualitative Sozialforschung*, 8, 2. http://nbn-resolving.de/urn:nbn:de:0114-fqs0702P75 (22 May 2022).

Reisigl, M. & Warnke, I. (2013). *Diskurslinguistik im Spannungsfeld von Deskription, Präskription und Kritik: Eine Einleitung.* In U.H. Meinhof, M. Reisigl & I. Warnke (eds.), Diskurslinguistik im Spannungsfeld von Deskription und Kritik (pp. 7–35). Berlin: Akademie Verlag.

Popper, R.K. (1994/1996). *In Search of a Better World: Lectures and Essays from Thirty Years.* London, New York: Routledge.

Russell, B. (1910). Knowledge by Acquaintance and Knowledge by Description. *Proceedings of the Aristotelian Society, 11*, 108–128. http://www.jstor.org/stable/4543805 (21 June 2022).

Spitzmüller, J., & Warnke, I. (2011). *Diskurslinguistik: Eine Einführung in Theorien und Methoden der transtextuellen Sprachanalyse.* Berlin, New York: De Gruyter.

Warnke, I.H. (ed.) (2007). *Diskurslinguistik nach Foucault: Theorien und Gegenstände.* Berlin, Boston: De Gruyter.

Wodak, R., Januschek, F., Czyżewski, M., House, J., & Duszak, A. (2010). Perspektiven der Kritischen Sozialwissenschaften im Allgemeinen und der Kritischen Diskursanalyse im Speziellen. In A. Duszak, J. House & Ł. Kumięga (eds.), *Globalization, Discourse, Media: In a Critical Perspective* (pp. 559–596). Warszawa: Wydawnictwa Uniwersytetu Warszawskiego.

Wodak, R. (2017). Kritische Diskursforschung. *Der Deutschunterricht*, *6*, 54–63.

Małgorzata Godlewska

Discursive Strategies in Anti-COVID-19 Vaccine Online Publications: A Case Study

Abstract

This research paper intends to investigate the discursive patterning of online publications collected from Joseph Mercola's official webpage devoted to promoting a healthy lifestyle and natural medicine. The qualitative study of a corpus of twenty-one publications, appearing since the pandemic period of COVID-19 till now, relies on the dialectical-relational approach to Critical Discourse Analysis, and resorts to the analytical method of discourse analysis proposed by Norman Fairclough (2003) as well as Eve Chiapello and Norman Fairclough (2013).

The analysis strives to map out recurrent discursive techniques relying on the tripartite model of analysis consisting of *genre*, *discourse*, and *style* categories. The study intends to interpret and evaluate the intricate relations between the various categories which build the *Discourse* of the website, and to investigate this *Discourse* as part of the social order which it addresses and as the manifestation of the constitution of the author's, i. e. Mercola's, social identity. The conclusions of this research hope to contribute to the discussion on the development of online crisis communication, particularly the anti-vaccine discourse in American society.

Keywords: critical discourse analysis, dialectical-relational approach, anti-vaccine discourse, conversationalisation of online discourse, anti-state discourse.

1. Introduction

The COVID-19 pandemic has exerted a tremendous impact on human lives and on people's consciousness worldwide. Despite the official anti-virus precautions and scientific evidence recommending the use of anti-COVID-19 vaccines promoted by the World Health Organisation and governmental health-care institutions, anti-vaccine rhetoric has been spreading through a variety of traditional news sources and online social media. The Centre for Countering Digital Hate, an American nonprofit organisation, submitted a list of twelve people "responsible

Małgorzata Godlewska, University of Gdansk, ORCID: 0000-0002-3425-4899.

for sharing 65 percent of all anti-vaccine messaging on social media", with Joseph Mercola occupying a number-one placement among other activists such as Robert F. Kennedy Jr. and the founder of the website Health Nut News, Erin Elizabeth, Mercola's life partner (Frenkel, 2021, para. 7). Mercola and his team have generated a wide array of anti-COVID-19 vaccine statements in the form of online publications on Mercola's website, Facebook and in their appearances on YouTube and Twitter. The popularity of Mercola's anti-vaccine activity has granted him about 1,7 million followers on the American Facebook page and around one million followers on the Spanish-language page (Frenkel, 2021, para. 22). Besides, the anti-vaccine policy conducted by Mercola's group is strictly linked to the promotion of his natural health business, at present amounting to $100 million (Frenkel, 2021, para. 22).

It is the intention of this paper to indicate and interpret the distinct features of the Discourse created on Mercola's official website which helped its founder to become a powerful anti-governmental figure and a guru among anti-COVID-19 vaccine communities. The analysis will involve the study of twenty-one articles published on Mercola's website in the years 2021–2023, all of which share an anti-COVID-19 vaccine attitude and embody Mercola's anti-government stance. The investigation into the corpus of online publications will involve a critical discourse perspective and will resort to Norman Fairclough's (2003) as well as Eve Chiapello and Norman Fairclough's (2013) research strategies in the analysis of discourses (2013). This research will try to detect and analyse discursive elements interspersed into the website publications together with the implications that these elements might entail for their readers. Hence, a qualitative analysis will be employed to display the types of recurrent discursive techniques in the corpus selected for the analysis. The results of the study are intended to reveal ideology hidden in the constructed narrative and hint at corporate goals which might underlie Mercola's anti-vaccine ideology.

2. Critical discourse analysis: background information and main approaches

The earliest attempts to investigate a text from the perspective of a textual unit longer than a sentence can be traced in the research of the 1960s and 70s and the publications of Terence F. Mitchell, Kenneth L. Pike, Michael Halliday, and Ruqaiya Hasan (Jaszczyk-Grzyb, 2021, 138). However, it is the research of such scholars as Teun A. van Dijk, Ruth Wodak, Anna Duszak, Norman Fairclough, as well as Lilie Chouliaraki and Norman Fairclough that paved the way towards the theoretical and practical development of CDA, that is Critical Discourse Analysis in the 1990s. Critical discourse analysis is grounded in the English critical linguistics of the 1970s, and it is indebted predominantly to three main theories: Western Marxism, Frankfurt's critical theory of Habermas and Foucault's theory of discourse (Duszak & Fairclough, 2008, 12). Norman Fairclough's *Language and Power* (1989) is regarded as a groundbreaking text, as Corsaro observes (1981, 854), which contributed significantly to the research in CDA, the scientific sub-discipline which seeks the relations between discourse and social elements such as ideology and power.

A vast number of scientific sub-disciplines can be indicated with a view to their shared interest in the issue of discourse, ranging over semiotics, pragmatics, psycho- and sociolinguistics, ethnography of speaking, conversation analysis, and discourse studies (Wodak & Meyer, 2015, 3). Besides, these subdisciplines coincide at seven points in their exploration of discourse and its paradigms and these include an interest in the "naturally occurring" language, the analytical focus on units larger than a word or a sentence, the study of language above the level of grammar to include interaction, the inclusion of non-verbal aspects of language and communication such as the visual, semiotic and multimodal aspects, the shift of interest towards the "dynamic socio-cognitive and interactional moves and strategies", "the study of functions of contexts of language use", the analysis of large aspects of text grammar and language use which include among others speech acts, politeness, interactions, coherence, topics, rhetoric which mark the text and discourse (Wodak & Meyer, 2015, 3). The aspect which differentiates discourse analysis from critical discourse analysis is, as Wodak and Meyer argue, the latter's problem-orientedness and the investigation of a linguistic unit from the social perspective through a multidisciplinary approach (2015, 3). It is a social phenomenon with the context of its use rather than an abstract linguistic unit which undergoes micro and macro-analysis.

It should be emphasised that CAD does not represent one theoretical school but is often defined as a range of approaches with different research paradigms. Norman Fairclough suggests a division of discourse analysis approaches, CAD being one of their versions, regarding a degree of detail in textual analysis (Fairclough, 2003, 3), which can be compared to the distinction of deductive and inductive approaches to discourse analysis proposed by Wodak and Meyer. Nevertheless, with a view to the central features of CDA such as its dynamicity and flexibility, the division between approaches should not be perceived as fixed but alternating during the entire process of social and textual analysis (Maghlouth, 2017, 20). Selected approaches to CDA are to be briefly outlined with particular attention paid to the dialectical-relational approach as the key tenet for the interpretation of the analytical material in this research paper.

The inductive approach involves a detailed case study to map out regular patterns in utterances, the strategy which can be identified in the research within the discourse-historical approach, corpus linguistics approach, social actors' approach, and dispositive analysis (Wodak & Meyer, 2015, 4). The discourse-historical approach to CDA, represented by Ruth Wodak and Martin Reisigl's research practice, focuses on the discourse model with specific conceptual tools, rather than on theories. Nevertheless, it is possible to discern the impact of grand linguistic theories such as argumentation theory, Halliday's systemic-functional theory of language or the socio-philosophical turn in critical theories (Jaszczyk-Grzyb, 2021, 162–163). Besides, since historical analysis is central to this approach, it is not surprising that politics and the political discourse it generates constitute the main targets of the DHA's scholars (Wodak & Meyer, 2015, 26). In addition, the concepts of "discursive elements" and "discursive strategies" are fundamental in the analysis of racist and antisemitic discourses (Jaszczyk-Grzyb, 2021, 163).

Wodak and Meyer accentuate the significance of the second approach mentioned, specifically, the corpus linguistics approach regarded by Wodak and Meyer as an advantageous extension to all the other CDA approaches (2015, 26). The techniques offered by the "corpus-assisted critical discourse analysis" or "corpus-assisted discourse research", the terms used to designate CDA interlinked with corpus linguistics, subvert criticism directed at CDA rooted in the subjectivity in the selection of research material and the lack of its representativeness and offer practical research tools, such as the use of frequency lists, the analysis of keyword lists, collocation lists or concordances (Jaszczuk-Grzyb, 2021, 177–183).

A different approach is proposed by Theo van Leeuwen and the Social Actors Approach, which also exemplifies an inductive strategy for the analysis of discourse. Its general framework hinges on Foucault's notion of discourse, which is established through the action of individual actors who "permanently reproduce social structure" (Wodak & Meyer, 2015, 27), thus connecting the sociological and linguistic theories. Discourse is defined as "recontextualization of social practice" (van Leeuwen, 2009, 148), while the study of social actors' discourses is intended to reveal and evaluate the degree of power exercised through their discourses. Linguistic parameters belong to the centre of investigation within this approach.

The sociocognitive and the dialectical–relational approaches share a deductive perspective due to their common analytical method, which focuses on the textual level rather than the linguistic surface of the collected data (Wodak & Meyer, 2015, 22). The sociocognitive approach is attributed to the work of Teun van Dijk, who postulated the use of the term Critical Discourse Studies instead of CDA to emphasise the variety of analytical methods and approaches which contribute to the field. Van Dijk specifies the central features of critical discourse analysis which encompass the focus on social problems and political issues in their contexts, its multidisciplinary quality, the analytical rather than merely descriptive aspect of CDS, and the goal of CDS to explore in detail how discursive structures legitimise and maintain the relations of domination in society (van Dijk, 2001, 353). The feature which should be highlighted concerning this approach is van Dijk's interpretation of discourse as a communicative event, thus incorporating various semiotic and multimodal elements apart from a written text into its definition.

The final dialectical-relational approach to CDA can be identified with a broad linguistic operationalisation and the emphasis placed on the discourse structure rather than on the agency in the process of discourse analysis (Wodak & Meyer, 2015, 22). Represented by Norman Fairclough, the approach is indebted to "grand" theories of Marx, Foucault, Bourdieu and Halliday analysing various forms of social change and "social wrongs", such as "injustice, inequality, lack of freedom" (Fairclough, 2013, 231), the use of power and resistance to it, and aiming to detect their reflections in discourse. The main goal of CDA from the dialectical-relational perspective rests on the study of "linguistic, semiotic and 'interdiscursive features of 'texts', inclusive of written documents as well as websites or interviews, which are part of processes of social change, but in ways which facilitate the productive integration of textual analysis into multi-disciplinary research on change" (Fairclough, 2001, 1–3).

Fairclough distinguishes a set of categories to be applied to the analysis of the dialectical relations between discourse and the social world. He understands social practices as "durable forms of social activity" which underlie specific fields and organisations, and which can include, though are not reducible to, elements such as activities, social relations, objects, instruments, time and place, social subjects with their beliefs, knowledge and values as well as semiosis (Fairclough, 2001, 2–3). All these relations are dialectically related and require analysis which would address other disciplines rather than merely a linguistic or solely social perspective, thus promoting a "transdisciplinary" analytical approach. Networks of social practices on their semiotic level result in the formation of "an order of discourse," specified by its inherent correlation of "genres," "discourses", and "styles" (Fairclough, 2003, 220).

Genres can be defined as "diverse ways of (inter)acting in their specifically semiotic aspect" (Fairclough, 2001, 4). Fairclough (2013, 214–216) differentiates distinct levels of genres, including *pre-genres*, for instance, Narrative and Report, secondly, "disembedded genres" and "situated genres", which are defined by their social practice, e.g. meetings, interviews, and news articles. The second category, specifically *discourses*, is equated with many ways of representing the social world attributed to a particular social group and their social practices, e.g. the poor, the government, or medicine, and involves a thorough linguistic textual analysis. *Style* is distinguished as the third category of an order of discourse indicative of a social agent's identity and ingrained in semiosis. The interdiscursive analysis of discourses involves the study of relations between orders of discourse to identify the semiotic difference in the process of making meaning and to assess the degree of dominance inscribed within particular discourses (Fairclough, 2001, 4). Thus, the linguistic and semiotic analysis of various texts belonging to selected orders of discourse is related to the context of particular social events and practices to reveal either innovative or conventional textual features, which mark the orders of discourse under the analysis.

Despite differences among the theoretical approaches mentioned, all the critical discourse research is preoccupied with the problem of social manipulation through language and with the conceptualisation of language as the medium of domination and social force, as Wodak and Meyer argue (2015, 13). Besides, the thematic preoccupations of CDA can range from the issues of globalisation, neoliberalism, climate change, ideologies, the government, "hegemonic struggles to give a "universal" status to particular discourses and representations", quoting Fairclough (2003, 7), who adds social change, change in communication technologies as well as "societal informalization" (ibid.: 7) to the list of contemporary social research topics which inspire scholars within critical discourse.

3. Methodology

This research involves the study of twenty-one online publications which appeared on Mercola's official website (www.mercola.com) in the years 2021–2023. Part of the publications had been downloaded from Mercola's website before 2022, after which date all the open-access articles related to COVID-19 were officially banned and, for this reason, transferred to the "censored private library", a distinct webpage which requires a paid subscription. The publications selected for the analysis were extracted either from the main web page or the censored private library database with the keyword search of "vaccine." Special attention was paid to the online material, which focuses on the issue of anti-Covid vaccine. The publications included in the corpus analysed have been labelled as Text 1–21, and their references are provided at the end of this paper under the section, "Internet sources: Joseph Mercola's publications".

The online publications were collected and investigated using Chiapello and Fairclough's tri-partite analytical model (2013) according to the aspects of *genre*, *style* and *discourse*, whose mutual relations texture one unique *Discourse* which transpires from the analysed corpus of texts. These mutual relations between the aspects of genre, discourse, and style are discussed to unveil the repetitive patterns texturing the *Discourse* generated by the publications extracted from the website. It is argued that the website can be regarded as a *Discourse* with a capital

"D" at an elevated level of abstraction, which can be perceived as a "configuration of discourses spelled with a lowercase 'd'" (Chiapello & Fairclough, 2013, 263). The analysis of the various configurations of semiotic elements and their patterning on the web page is intended to inform about the methods of discourse formation and about the ideology which underlies the creation of the Discourse of Mercola's website.

4. The analysis of Mercola's website: the networking of genres, discourses, and styles

4.1. Genres

Fairclough does not provide a clear definition of genre and genre classification but, instead, he distinguishes between *pre-genres, disembedded genres* and *situated genres* (2003, 68). Viewed from this perspective, the corpus of selected publications manifests a hybrid generic structure established by the main genre markers of the pre-genre of argument and the secondary genre markers of a promotional brochure of Mercola's healthcare online store. The latter exemplifies a *situated genre*, which is a genre "specific for particular purposes" (Fairclough, 2003, 69), which in the context of the analysed publications can be attributed to marketing.

Concerning the structure of the pre-genre of argument, notably a problem-solution argument, it is claimed that all of the texts discussed display an overall framework common to academic research papers with headings and subheadings signalling the essential thematic concerns of the paper and manifesting the anti-COVID-19 vaccine perspective directly or implicitly. Almost all of the main headings use the central concept of anti-COVID-19 vaccine adjacent to a linguistic unit which triggers negative associations, such as "scare" and "harassment" in Text 6, "original antigenic sin" and "the hidden danger of Covid shots", "boosting may backfire", "covid jabs… excess deaths" in Text 9, "disturbing evidence" and "covid shots… too late to recover" in Text 10, "jabs may raise risk of Covid death", "Covid shots kill brain and heart cells", "covid shots can kill" in Text 12, "Covid jab does more harm than good" in Text 14. The lexeme of death is reiterated through the majority of analysed publications either in the main heading or in the sub-headings, manifesting the author's general critical stance towards the anti-COVID policy and alarming the readers about the problem's saliency due to the frequency of its application in the texts.

The compositional elements of the pre-genre of argument are reflected in the structure of the analysed texts and include an abstract, entitled "Story At-A-

Glance", which incorporates the main thematic issues in the form of a series of bulleted statements, a brief introduction which partly covers the contents of the abstract, paragraphs delineating a research problem, its origins, and development, and a current situation related to the problem analysed. Each publication is supported with references to secondary sources which include scientific reviews, government databases, such as Florida or California bills, WHO announcements and recommendations, news, and interviews with representatives of the anti-Covid vaccine viewpoint including medical doctors (dr Aseem Malhorta in Text 2), researchers (dr Paul Marik in Text 15), journalists (WhatsHerFace in Text 2), and politicians (Robert F. Kennedy Jr. in Text 3).

Concluding remarks contained in the final part of the publications often incorporate a paragraph devoted to instructions on anti-COVID-19 prevention, a warning against anti-COVID-19 vaccine, promotion of early anti-COVID-19 treatment with the aid of natural medicine, as well as treatments offered by Mercola's online shop and by medical institutions which he supports, as in Texts 1, 2, 5, 12, 18 and 21. These thematic issues indicate the presence of genre markers of a promotional brochure, also manifested graphically by the commercial of Mercola's natural medicine store.

Despite the common framework of an academic research paper, the publications do not include the clear scientific methodology used for the analysis of research questions devoted to the anti-COVID-19 vaccine or other co-related issues which would underlie the arguments forwarded in the texts. Besides, the selection of the resources might also be regarded as debatable since the author relies primarily on opinions expressed by popular anti-COVID-19 vaccine opponents, such as Robert F. Kennedy Jr. in Text 3, or proponents of alternative medicine instead of the conventional medical treatments, such as, for instance, Vladimir Zelenko in Text 1, renowned for the "unfounded treatment" for COVID-19 officially disclaimed by American researchers (Risen, 2022).

The genre mixture observed within the analytical corpus of texts can be analysed concerning the purpose of a given genre or genre chain, the idea which may not be accentuated, though (Fairclough, 2003, 70–86). Fairclough uses Habermas's distinction between "communicative" actions, i. e. interactions which focus on understanding, and "strategic" actions, interactions which lead towards getting results (2003, 71). Mercola's publications manifest a hybrid of communicative and strategic actions, manifested through the genre mixture of an argument of the "problem-solution" type, and the subsidiary genre of a brochure, which promotes non-conventional medicine, such as vitamin C and D or nebulised peroxide advertised in Text 1 (2021). The goals of the website include both aims: the communicative aim of informing the readers about a healthy lifestyle obtained with the aid of natural medicine offered by Mercola's online store, and the implied strategic aim of the marketing text. The subgenre of a promotional brochure is best exemplified by the final seven paragraphs in Text 1 (2021), which promote the use of hydrogen peroxide and vitamin C to prevent COVID-19 and urge the reader to visit Mercola's online store.

Because genres are manifested on two levels, the semantic and the lexico-grammatical ones (Fairclough, 2021), it is necessary to discuss the corpus of publications with a view to their leitmotifs and the frequency of their appearance. The set of central themes relies on the list proposed by Liu et al. (2022) and includes the first eight basic categories proposed by the authors and two additional ones (9 and 10), added to this analytical corpus. The themes include: 1. A clinical trial or test of vaccines, 2. The authorisation of vaccines, 3. The safety of vaccines, 4. The approval of vaccines, 5. The development and production of vaccines, 6. Vaccine's effects in preventing symptoms of COVID-19 illness, 7. Vaccines proved as promising, 8. Efficacy of vaccines, 9. The government's anti-COVID-19 vaccine policy, 10. An after-COVID-19 dystopian vision of humanity. Mercola's publications of 2021, represented by Texts 1–4 centre around the issues of safety and efficacy of vaccines, the vaccine's effects in preventing COVID-19 (dominant themes in texts 1, 2, 3), and the clinical trial or test (dominant themes in texts: 2, 3, 4). Text 4 diverges from the other publications since its central themes include the authorisation of vaccines, the development and production of vaccines as well as the government's anti-COVID-19 policy. The theme of the development and production appears a few times in Texts 2 and 4 together with the theme of the government's anti-COVID-19 vaccine policy mentioned in Text 1.

The second group of fifteen publications which appeared in 2022 outnumbers the other two sets, thus reflecting an increased interest in the issue of anti-COVID-19 vaccination. The first four texts in this group (Texts 5–8) and Texts 11, 13, and 15 share the focus on the issue of the government's anti-vaccine policy in the USA and in the world. The same theme constitutes a secondary issue, though still emphasised as valid, in publications 9 and 14. The themes which seem to be reiterated through almost all 2022 publications include the safety of vaccines (Texts: 5, 8, 9, 10, 13, 14, 15), vaccine's effects in preventing COVID-19 (Texts: 12, 14, and, as a secondary theme, in Texts 5, 9, 10, 15) and the efficacy of vaccines (Texts: 12, 14, 9, 10). The publications of 2022 bring new subjects to Mercola's website such as the issue of clinical trials and testing discussed in Texts 5, 8, 9, 10, and 14. The theme of the after-COVID-19 vision of humanity from a dystopian perspective constitutes a secondary issue in publications 8 and 13.

The final group of publications of 2023 returns to the topics of the safety of vaccines (Texts: 17, 18, 19, 20) and the effects of vaccines in preventing COVID-19 (Texts: 17, 18, 19, 21). The themes echoing in this set also include the government's anti-COVID-19policy (Texts: 16, 18, 19) and the efficacy of vaccines (Texts: 17, 18, 19). The other themes raised in publications of this period (Texts 19 and 20) include the interest in clinical trials and testing the authorisation of vaccines (Texts 19, 20), as well as the approval of vaccines.

The study of all the thematic issues which appeared on the webpage during the period 2021–2023 reveals the lack of publications or passages within publications devoted to the presentation of anti-COVID-19 vaccines from a positive angle. Thus, the omission of category seven, i. e. "vaccines proved as promising", must be recognised as a significant and conscious determinant of the thematic profile of Mercola's webpage. What is more, the increased frequency of the theme of the government's anti-COVID-19 vaccine policy in the set of 2022 can be attributed partly to a cyberattack on Mercola's website, the event described by Mercola in Text 7 and attributed by the webpage's author to the government's unfounded interference.

Furthermore, the thematic issues common to the texts published in 2023 differ from the earlier sets in their primary focus: while the early texts devote attention to the analysis of vaccines with a view to their safety, efficacy, and side effects, the latter ones treat these aspects as unarguable and can be equated with a co-text, i. e. common knowledge resources shared between the author and the readers. This co-text might be used to trigger assumptions about the latest threats to civilisation, such as a new anti-COVID-19 vaccine against recent COVID variants, e. g. Omicron mentioned in Text 19, post-jab deaths caused by two anti-COVID-19 vaccines (Text 18), chronic obstructive pulmonary disease (Text 17), and iDNA vaccines as a new type of gene therapy vaccines derived from the anti-COVID-19 prototype (Text 21). All of these newly observed threats to human existence, in a similar vein as the early anti-COVID-19 vaccine and all the pandemic restrictions, contribute to the creation of a dystopian vision of "transhumanism" under the guise of medical experiments and according to the dictate of the "Big-Pharma" corporations, billionaires such as Bill Gates and the US government officials, including the president Joe Biden, all representatives of the conspiracy theories discussed in Texts 7, 8 and 10 of 2022, at the time of the ban imposed on Mercola's website.

4.2. Discourses and styles

The Discourse of Mercola's website transpires from a network of discourses, specifically the connectionist and inspirational ones interlaced with the discourse of a medical expert, the anti-governmental discourse, and the promotional discourse, which can be distinguished by their ways of representing social aspects of reality on the levels of vocabulary, semantic relations, and grammar. The constitution of the authorial identity within one global Discourse on the website can be claimed to be implemented through texturing the relations of equivalence and difference observed predominantly on the level of style, lexis, and grammar.

The Discourse in all the publications under the analysis is textured by a mixture of formal and informal registers where conversational English coincides with medical terms and formal grammatical structures. However, most paragraphs containing specialised medical registers constitute quotes from secondary specialised sources rather than from Mercola's scientific work. Text 1 (2021) summarises the research conducted by Vladimir Zelenko, a medical doctor and a famous anti-vaxxer, and manifests the high-low register clash which defines the style of the publications:

> So, on that note, Zelenko and I take a deep dive into what can be done to prevent such a fate. Zelenko categorizes the risks of COVID-19 "vaccines" into three categories: acute, subacute and long-term, so let's begin by reviewing the primary risks found in each of these categories. The acute phase of harm begins at the moment of injection and likely lasts for about three months or so. Based on reports filed with the U.S. Vaccine Adverse Event Reporting System (VAERS), it's clear that many cannot survive past the acute phase. About 6,000 deaths have been reported so far.... (Text 1, 2021, para. 5)

The informal sentence structure at the beginning of the quote, "so, on that note," and conversational English exemplified by the idiomatic phrase "take a deep dive" are contrasted with the categories of risks enumerated in the second sentence. Moreover, the contrast is strengthened by the formal structures of the final sentences (e.g. Based on reports ... have been reported) as well as a more sophisticated vocabulary, exemplified by the words "acute" and "subacute phase". Mercola quotes Zelenko's research paper, written in formal scientific English, and summarises Zelenko's report in a formal and specialised register, though interspersed with colloquial structures, as in the passage: "As the **mRNA** disseminates through your vascular system, the cells lining your blood vessels begin producing **spike proteins**. This is why we're seeing such a staggering number of reports of people experiencing **blood clots** from these injections" (Text 1, 2021, para. 12). The underlined phrases, graphically highlighted in the original text, as well as the other lexical units such as "disseminates", "vascular system" "blood vessels" manifest sophisticated vocabulary typical of medical research papers, though interrupted by the informality and directness of tone found in the initial part of the sentence "This is why we're seeing...".

The technique of juxtaposing high versus low registers on the level of lexis and grammar constitutes a prevalent technique in all the analysed publications. This signals a conscious tendency leading towards the informalisation of the style of the publications, which represent primarily a formal pre-genre of argument, and the medical discourse. As a result of this stylistic strategy, the distance in the relations between the author-reader and the expert-layperson is diminished.

Besides, the publications of late 2022 and 2023 show the growing intensity of conversationalisation and the emotional load of narration on the stylistic and lexical language levels. Text 20 (2023) begins the introduction using a highly informal style with a direct appeal to the readers, as in the line, "If you thought mRNA injections were the craziest things the vaccine industry has cooked up lately, you haven't seen the half of it yet. Up next, we have so-called "immunization DNA" or iDNA," a novel class of gene therapy "vaccines" … (Text 20, 2023, para. 6). The informal register is intensified by the use of emotional defining elements, such as the adjective "craziest" and the phrasal verb "cooked up", the use of contracted forms, e. g. "haven't", and an ironic lexical element, "so-called" used to define a formal medical term, "immunization" belonging to a specialised scientific jargon. The same publication inserts emotional and informal phrases before or after scientific and formal quotes from medical research papers, such as the following, "Oh joy. Considering the shocking harms mRNA injections are causing…" (Text 20, 2023, para: 19). Other examples of informal structures include units such as interjections "so" and "well" and a conjunction "but" used at the beginning of sentences following medical narration, as in the example, "So, just how would an iDNA shot affect just "a small number of cells"…" (Text 20, 2023, para: 22) and expressions of exaggeration and sarcasm, as in the line, "Never mind the fact that never-before-seen "turbo cancers" are sending people to their graves in record numbers. Nothing to see there" (Text 20, 2023, para: 43).

The application of the plural pronoun "we" might be claimed to be an indicator of the author's attempt to decrease the distance in the social relations between the author-expert and the reader and build a connectionist discourse. The selection of the plural pronoun with the technique of juxtaposing high versus low registers might be perceived as a cognizant strategy intended to include the author, i. e. Mercola, into the group of his readers, thus diminishing their mutual distance. The application of the first-person pronouns is visible in the set of publications of 2022 and, though to a lower degree, in the set of 2023.

Mercola's texts clearly define the social relations between the antagonists and protagonists, placing the author beside the readers. In Text 15 (2022), Mercola speaks of himself in the first person in the section "The Hunt for Truth-Tellers" where he depicts his anti-vaccine attitude and his open engagement in the anti-governmental and anti-vax activity, "I've written several articles over the past couple of years detailing the brutal and unethical treatment of medical professionals who have dared to speak out against any part of the irrational COVID narrative" (ibid. para. 49). In the closing section, the author directs an appeal to the readers where he places himself next to other medical doctors and the protagonists of his anti-vaccine publications, "if you or someone you know still cannot believe that a doctor would ever withhold information or straight out a lie to you, listen to Kirsch's interview with Marik. Listen to Nass's story. Reda Kory's book. Look at the legislation being pushed through in California" (ibid. para. 72). The quotation leads to assumptions about the categorisation of "antagonists" among the governmental institutions and "the protagonists" among doctors and himself. The author directly addresses the culprits of the COVID pandemic including the state and its institutions, such as AMA accused of "lawlessness" (Text 15, 2022, para. 66), "Big Pharma" placed neighbouring the term "propaganda" in a single phrase (Text 15, 2022, para. 68), California bureaucrats "violating the U.S. Constitution and destroying the medical profession ... pushing medical science back into the Dark Age" (Text 15, 2022, para. 68), because of censoring his website for misinformation.

Apart from the direct accusations against the antagonists indicated above, Mercola's publications try to bring the author into a more personal relationship with the readers through using the first person pronouns *I* and *we* together, as in the line, "To them, you and I are not only ignorant and contemptible but a resource to be used and disposed of at will… They intend to seize complete control over the world and implement tyrannical global slavery, and to do that, they have to silence any and all opposition… I am committed to continue to empower you with the truth about health and the global cabal's threats to your health and liberty" (para. 16–17). Thus, the text presents the author and the reader as victims of the same system threatening human freedom. It should be stressed that every paragraph in this section of the publication "The Soul and Freedom of Humanity Is at Stake" begins with pronouns which specify social relations between the readers and the author, e.g.: "I've discussed…" (para. 1), "To them…", "you and I…" (para. 2), "They intend to seize control…" (para. 3), "No matter what they throw at us, we simply must stay the course…" (para. 4), "I am committed to empower you…" (para. 5). The first-person pronouns create a regular structure of the text and attract the reader's attention. The style relies on a personal and emotional tone and informal or neutral vocabulary. This emotional address to the readers and the direct and friendly appeal constitutes a recurrent rhetorical device in several publications in the final section (Text 1, 2021; Text 2, 2021; Text 5, 2022; Text 9, 2022; Text 19, 2023; Text 21, 2023; Text 20, 2023; Text 18, 2023). This discursive strategy consequently textures the connectionist discourse in the medical discourse found in the publications.

The inspirational and connectionist discourses transpire from Mercola's emotional narration, intensified by stylistic devices, such as metaphors and similes. The strategy might be directed towards further informalisation of Mercola's narration in the publications, in contrast to the formal and impersonal language of the publications from governmental institutions and research material. Furthermore, Mercola's Discourse attempts to establish a strong bond between the website's creator and his followers through references to the shared system of ethical values and convictions which are claimed to be grounded in the high regard for freedom, since, as Mercola argues, "Standing up for a good cause – and there's no better cause than freedom – actually makes you more powerful" and, in another line, "We simply cannot give up our rights and freedom" – for any reason – because they won't stop there" (Text 7, 2022, pars. 27–30). Rhetorical devices applied on the website manage to texture equivalence relations between the author and the readers and shape contrastive relations between the readers, inclusive of the author, and the state and pharmaceutical business. These relations can be argued as responsible for generating inspirational and connectionist discourses, using Boltanski and Chiapello's terms (Fairclough, 2013, 272).

The majority of the analysed publications construct the connectionist discourse relying on the antagonist-protagonist relations which underlie the publications employing the metaphor of war. The repetitive rhetorical figure is employed to represent the pandemic realms, with the concept of vaccine and vaccination lying at the centre. It should be highlighted that the term *vaccine* appears predominantly in the paragraphs quoted from scientific medical journals and official government announcements. In the publication sections filtered through the author's perspective, either presented in his own words or through an interviewee's narration, the word *vaccine* is replaced with a *shot* or *jab*. The first term prevails in the early publications of 2021 and is used alternately with a *jab* in the later publications. Nevertheless, the lexeme *jab*, more informal than *vaccine*, significantly outnumbers the other terms in the set of texts of 2022 and 2023. The definite preference for the informal term over the formal one enhances the impression of conversationalisation of the narration on the website, and the formulation of negative associations provoked by the word *jab*, defined in the Webster's Dictionary as "a quick thrust, blow, or punch" (1997, 722) in contrast to a neutral and scientific term *vaccine*.

Apart from the words *shot* and *jab* to designate anti-COVID vaccine, the author applies a range of metaphorical expressions which carry pejorative connotations, such as "bioweapons" (Text 10), "crime" (Text 19, 11) and "the riskiest and deadliest injections" (Text 8) and "Zyklon-V" (Text 1). The use of vaccination is compared to "an assault on your body" (Text 18, 20), "immune imprinting", and "handcuffs" on your immune system (Text 9). The pandemic is compared by the author to "war" (Text 1, 5, 7, 14) and "war against God" (Text 1), "a crusade" (Text 7), "global cabal" (Text 7), "massacre" (Text 21), "the global takeover" (Text 19), "calamity" and "madness" (Text 20), "the carnage" (Text 14), and, quoting other critics' words, "perfect set up for genocide" and "weapon of mass destruction" (Text 1). Hospitals are presented as "killing fields" where "reckless authorities" "push people" to use vaccines and where doctors "are deceiving" patients who, compared to "cash cows," are "tortured and killed" (Text 15).

Another repetitive metaphorical conceptualisation of the pandemic is triggered by phraseology related to religious conflicts, exemplified by the phrases, a "witch hunt" for "truth-tellers" (Text 15), "pushing medical science back to Dark Ages" (Text 15), "the original antigenic sin of vaccine" (Text 9), "madness", "something horrific … killing people" and "deaths piling up by the day" (Text 14). The anti-vaxxers are labelled as "brave hearts" and "heroes" (Text 15) hunted for speaking the truth against the "death cult gospel" (Text 10) in the times of the global "conspiracy" leading towards "the era of transhumanism" (Text 20) and "human augmentation" (Text 20). The catastrophic vision of the future depicted in Mercola's narration includes "cornucopia of mRNA shots" (Text 20) which are "in control of brain function" (Text 20). He claims to speak for "millions [of people who] will die in the murderous cabal" of "forcing drugs under the threat of death" (Text 20). The Discourse strengthened by these metaphors appeals to human emotions and might trigger associations with the persecution of minority groups officially condemned by the controlling system. Through references to the co-text, which is the shared knowledge resources, the readers and the author are positioned as equal but in opposition to the controlling American healthcare institutions which impose the anti-COVID-19 vaccine. Thus, the inspirational discourse of shared negative emotions contributes to the generation of the connectionist discourse between the readers and the author.

The use of the repetitive conceptual metaphor in the corpus of texts is diversified in the three groups of publications and ranges from rare in the first set of 2021 to very frequent in the group of texts published in 2022 and 2023. The metaphor of war which textures publications of 2022 relies on strong emotional language and equates the pandemic and vaccine with the worst world historical events. In contrast, the metaphorical representation of the pandemic in the texts of 2023 resorts to futuristic images through concepts such as transhumanism, experiments with human bodies, and the world conspiracy theory blaming the billionaires and the state for controlling people to gain power and riches, the idea clearly stated in Text 16 and manifested by the heading "COVID Advances New World Order – The Empire of Billionaires" (Text 7, 9, 21, 19).

It might be claimed that the publications of 2023 and partly of 2022 represent a new form of discourse gradually built upon the medical expert discourse of the early publications and formulated on the grounds of the initial connectionist and inspirational discourses. The new anti-governmental discourse expresses a confident narrative voice of an anti-vaxxer. This discourse gains prominence over the medical discourse since it is built on the anti-vaccine co-text of the previous publications, as in Text 20, "If you thought mRNA injections were the craziest things the vaccine industry has cooked up lately, you haven't seen half of it yet" (para. 6) and in Text 18, "Disturbingly, but not surprisingly, they [experts] concluded that 62.5% to 73.9% of post-jab deaths were likely caused by the injection" (para.7). The elements underlined belong to the readers' prior awareness of the assumed inefficacy and the risks of taking anti-COVID-19 vaccines, formulated in Mercola's texts and textured into their shared knowledge resources.

Apart from the expert and the anti-state discourses, the publications manifest the presence of the promotional discourse created by a successful businessperson with the strategic aim of advertising Mercola's website store. All the publications belonging to the analytical corpus contain passages devoted to the promotion of natural medicine products and therapies, part of which can be found in Mercola's online store located on the website. The promotional sections of the narration contain either the same or similar statements which warn against the anti-COVID-19 vaccine, popularise alternative therapies and Mercola's products, and advertise the website store and Mercola's anti-government activities. Text 1 opens with a section "a story at-a-glance" and the summary of negative effects of vaccines as well as a promotion of the following products: vitamins D and C, zinc, a zinc ionophore, NAC, a tabletop jet nebulizer, saline solution, food grade hydrogen peroxide (pars. 1–4). Text 2 places the information about alternative treatments at the end of the publication under the heading "Alternative Treatments" which includes "nebulized hydrogen peroxide for prevention and treatment of COVID-19". Text 12 lists a number of "other helpful treatments and remedies", the quote constitutes the heading from the publication, and contains e.g. "hyperbaric oxygen therapy", "time-restricted eating", and "pharmaceutical grade methylene blue", which is claimed to help "those suffering from long-haul COVID" since its ingredient "has been used to treat malaria since 1890" (pars. 67–73). Text 21 of 2023 inserts a few passages promoting "spike protein detox" with the aid of two drugs, "hydroxychloroquine and ivermectin" for those "injured by the COVID jab" (pars. 57–61). A similar set of paragraphs can be detected at the end of Text 20 of 2023 under the same heading "Resources for those injured by the COVID jab".

All the publications of the corpus successfully intertwine the elements of the medical expert discourse with the promotional discourse to connect the communicative aim of narration with the strategic one. The antagonist-protagonist social relations created within the discourses of the medical expert and the anti-governmental discourse contribute to the generation of the connectionist and inspirational discourses which can be claimed to lie at the foundation of the general Discourse rooted in the social identity of the author.

5. Conclusions

The website structure creates a semblance of open communication, a live debate on serious medical and governmental issues between Mercola, a medical doctor, a specialist, and a real-life person, rather than an anonymous institution such as the government itself, and an average citizen. The website can be compared to what Fairclough labels as a contemporary genre for "action at a distance", "genres of governance (…) through which organizations communicate with individuals (…) pervasively characterized by simulated social relations which, we might argue, tend to mystify social hierarchy and social distance" (2003, 76).

Mercola's website might be claimed to represent a Discourse which successfully contests the official U.S. government's order of discourse through its anti-vaccine narration, just as any capitalist order can be "constantly traversed by critique" (Chiapello & Fairclough, 2013, 266). The analysis and interpretation of the online texts extracted from Mercola's website inform about the complex structure of the author's Discourse built upon a network of discourses: a scientific discourse of a medical expert, a promotional discourse of a businessman, a conspiracy discourse, an anti-governmental discourse and the connectionist and inspirational discourses as components of each of these types. Mercola's Discourse can be claimed to be textured through the intersection of all these discourses and founded on the principle of equivalence and difference, gradually consolidating the relationship between the readers–viewers of the website and its author.

The analysis of the publications reveals that all of them construct the global Discourse by the use of the central principle of equivalence and difference but applying divergent methods within the sets of publications. The texts which discuss the anti-COVID-19 vaccine issue and the pandemic exemplary of 2021 communicate the anti-COVID-19 vaccine narration using a mixture of formal and informal registers, though within the patterns of an academic style, and transcribe into the pre-genre of argument. The prevalent thematic issues include the safety and side effects of vaccines, though they are not limited to them: health care constitutes another dominant theme.

The study of the principle of equivalence and difference realised in the publications of 2022 and 2023 shows a gradual tendency towards strengthening the relationship between the readers and the author and deepening the gap between the protagonists, that is the readers and the author, and the government institutions and pharmaceutical companies whose stance is perceived as directed against the human rights to freedom and the freedom of expression in particular. The themes of publications include anti-governmental texts, and the anti-COVID-19 vaccine subject inevitably leads towards assumptions about the government's manipulation. The publications of 2023 attack the state for the involvement with the pharmaceutical corporations in the conspiracy against humanity in a direct manner. The anti-COVID-19 narration alters into the revolutionary anti-state discourse which abandons an initial attenuated semi-formal register for the sake of a more colloquial tone of narration which, in 2023, manifests the strong emotional engagement, rich figurative language and semi-informal register with direct accusations infrequently interrupted by disrespectful statements in the publications.

The Discourse functions as a practical tool in Mercola's social and business enterprises since it has been attracting hundreds of people to follow his online activities and popularising his website with online publications and a non-conventional medical treatment store. Mercola's Discourse has been recognised by the American authorities as the number one misinformation spreader, thus admitting the power of his narrative strategy, even though this power is frequently criticised for resorting to manipulation. The aspects of Mercola's narration which undermine his credibility as a social activist in the pandemic order of discourse include the lack of objectivism in the selection of publication material since all the texts published on his platform manifest only one side of the social problem, namely the one representing his perspective. Hence, the second seeming quality of his publications, which is dialogism stemming from intertextuality, must be viewed as limited and discriminatory.

Nevertheless, the central features of narration which allow Mercola to build his distinct Discourse encompass, first, the informalisation of language through the mixture of styles, registers, and genres which, as Fairclough argues (2003, 86), has the potential to simulate public conversational exchange; second, the semblance of intertextuality achieved through the inclusion of quotations from interviews, monologues and numerous secondary scientific sources and government databases; and, finally, the establishment of a solid and evolving reader–viewer–author relationship obtained through texturing his personal and social identities onto the semantic, lexical, and structural levels of his texts.

Works cited

Chiapello, E. & Fairclough, N. (2013). Understanding the New Management Ideology. A transdisciplinary Contribution from Critical Discourse Analysis and the New Sociology of Capitalism. In N. Fairclough (ed.), *Critical Discourse Analysis. The Critical Study of Language* (pp. 255–280). London, New York: Routledge.

Corsaro, W. (1981). Rev. of *Language and Control.* Fowler, R., Kress, G., Hodge, B. & Trew, T. (1979). London: Routledge and Kegan Paul. *Social Forces*, 59/3, 854–856. doi:10.1093/sf/59.3.854.

Van Dijk, T. (2001). Critical Discourse Analysis. In D. Tannen, H. Hamilton & D. Schiffrin (eds.), *The Handbook of Discourse Analysis* (pp. 352–371). Oxford: Blackwell.
Duszak, A. & Fairclough, N. (2008). *Krytyczna analiza dyskursu. Interdyscyplinarne podejście do komunikacji społecznej.* Kraków: Universitas.
Fairclough, N. (2013). *Critical Discourse Analysis. The Critical Study of Language.* London, New York: Routledge.
Fairclough, N. (2003). *Analysing Discourse. Textual Analysis for Social Research.* London, New York: Routledge.
Fairclough, N. (2001). Critical Discourse Analysis. https://www.researchgate.net/publication/281506450_Critical_Discourse_Analysis#fullTextFileContent (07 October 2023).
Frankel, S. (2021). The Most Influential Spreader of Coronavirus Misinformation Online – The New York Times. https://www.nytimes.com/2021/07/24/technology/joseph-mercola-coronavirus-Misinformation-online.html (24 July 2021).
Grzmil-Tylutki, H. (2010). *Francuska lingwistyczna teoria dyskursu: historia, tendencje, perspektywy.* Kraków: Universitas.
Jaszczyk-Grzyb, M. (2021). *Mowa nienawiści ze względu na przynależność etniczną i narodową w komunikacji internetowej.* Poznań: Wydawnictwo Naukowe UAM.
Liu M., Ruinan, Z. & Ngai, C. (2022). Vaccines, media, and politics: A corpus-assisted discourse study of press representations of the safety and efficacy of COVID-19 vaccines. *PLoSONE*, 17, 12. https://www.researchgate.net/publication/366712623_Vaccines_media_and_politics_A_corpusasisted_discourse_study_of_press_representations_of_the_safety_and_efficacy_of_COVID-19_vaccines#fullTextFileContent (12 November 2023).
Maghlouth, Shrouq Hamad A. (2017). Critical Discourse Analysis of Social Change in Women-related Posts on Saudi English-Language Blogs Posted between 2009 and 2012. https://www.researchgate.net/publication/361369164_A_Critical_Discourse_Analysis_of_Social_Change_in_Women-_related_Posts_on_Saudi_English-Language_Blogs_Posted_between_2009_and_2012 (07 October 2023).
Mercola, J. Website. https://www.mercola.com. (29 October 2023).
Risen, C. (2022). Vladimir Zelenko, 48, Dies; Promoted an Unfounded Covid Treatment. *The New York Times.* https://www.nytimes.com/2022/07/01/us/vladimir-zelenko-dead.html. (01 July 2023).
Van Leeuwen, T. (2009). Discourse as the recontextualization of social practice: A guide. In R. Wodak & M. Meyer (eds.), *Methods of critical discourse analysis*, 2nd edition (pp. 144–161). London: Sage.
Wodak R. & Meyer, M. (eds.) (2015). Critical Discourse Analysis: History, Agenda, Theory, and Methodology. Los Angeles, London, New Delhi, Singapore, Washington DC: Sage. https://www.researchgate.net/publication/284725833_Critical_discourse_studieshistory_agenda_theory_and_methodology> (24 September 2023).

Internet sources: Joseph Mercola's publications

(Text 1), Mercola, J. (2021). Might Covid Injections Reduce Lifespan. https://takecontrol.substack.com/p/covid-vaccine-risks?utm_source=%Search%Fcovid&utm_medium=reader2 (20 August 2023).

(Text 2), Mercola, J. (2021). Are Covid Shots Fueling More Dangerous Mutations?. https://takecontrol.substack.com/p/covid-shots-drive-mutations (09 July 2023).

(Text 3), Mercola, J. (2021). How the Covid-19 Vaccine Destroys Your Immune System, https://takecontrol.substack.com/p/coronavirus-antibody-dependent-enhancement. (12 August 2023).

(Text 4), Mercola, J. (2021). Covid-19: Moderna Gets Its Miracle. https://takecontrol.substack.com/p/covid-19-moderna-hail-mary-moment?utm_source=%2Fsearch%2fModerna%2520gets%2520its%2520miracle&utm_medium=reader2 (22 March 2023).

(Text 5), Mercola, J. (2022). The Truth is Coming Out About Covid Deaths. https://takecontrol.substack.com/p/covid-death-statistics. (04 August 2022).

(Text 6), Mercola, J. (2022). The Great Vaccine Scare Reaches Fever Pitch. https://takecontrol.substack.com/p/the-great-vaccine-scare?utm_source=%2Fsearch%2Fcovid%2520vaccin&utm_medium=reader2 (02 March 2023).

(Text 7), Mercola, J. (2022). Mercola Website Shutdown – Why You May Be Next. https://takecontrol.substack.com/p/mercola-website-shutdown (30 September 2022).

(Text 8), Mercola, J. (2022). Executive Order Advances Biotech-Transhumanist Agenda. https://takecontrol.substack.com/p/advancing-biotechnology-and-Biomanufacturing (30 October 2022).

(Text 9), Mercola, J. (2022). Original Antigenic Sin – The Hidden Danger of Covid Shots. https://takecontrol.substack.com/p/original-antigenic-sin-covid-19?utm_source=%2Fsearch%2fThe%2520original%2520antigenic%2520sin&utm_medium=reader2 (30 October 2022).

(Text 10), Mercola, J. (2022). Covid Jab mRNA Detected in Human Breastmilk. https://takecontrol.substack.com/p/mrna-vaccine-detected-in-human-breastmilk (12 December 2022).

(Text 11), Mercola J. (2022). Health Officials Admit Bill Gates Runs the World. https://takecontrol.substack.com/p/does-bill-gates-run-the-world (02 December 2022).

(Text 12), Mercola, J. (2022). The Trail of Blood From the COVID Jabs. https://takecontrol.substack.com/p/covid-vaccine-and-blood-clots (05 December 2022).

(Text 13), Mercola, J. (2022). New Communist Law Forces Doctors to Promote Pharma Products. https://takecontrol.substack.com/p/law-forces-doctors-to-promote-Pharma-product (03 December 2022).

(Text 14), Mercola, J. (2022). More Studies Confirm the COVID Jab Does More Harm Than Good. https://takecontrol.substack.com/p/covid-shots-cause-more-harm-than-good (04 December 2022).

(Text 15), Mercola, J. (2022). Why Doctors Are Lying to You. https://takecontrol.substack.com/p/why-doctors-are-lying-to-you (12 December 2022).

(Text 16), Mercola, J. (2023). COVID Advances New World Order – The Empire of Billionaires. https://takecontrol.substack.com/p/united-nations-and-new-world-order (02 March 2023).

(Text 17), Mercola, J. (2023). What Toxic Wildfires Can Teach Us About COPD and COVID-19. https://takecontrol.substack.com/p/wildfire-toxicity (09 September 2023).
(Text 18), Mercola, J. (2023). Study: 74% of Post-Jab Deaths Caused by the Shot. https://takecontrol.substack.com/p/post-covid-vaccination-deaths (20 October 2023).
(Text 19), Mercola, J. (2023). What You Need to Know About the Latest COVID Jab Rollout. https://takecontrol.substack.com/p/latest-covid-jab-rollout (10 November 2023).
(Text 20), Mercola, J. (2023). iDNA Vaccines to Generate Interna Virus Production. https://takecontrol.substack.com/p/idna-vaccines (25 November 2023).
(Text 21), Mercola, J. (2023). Are COVID Jab Deaths Being Covered Up? https://articles.mercola.com/sites/articles/archive/2023/11/25/covid-vaccine-deaths-cover-Up.aspx (26 November 2023).

Silvia Bonacchi

Haters in the Vaccination Conflict in Italy[1]: A Study of Selected Posts on Telegram, YouTube, Twitter and Facebook

Abstract
What forms does hate speech take in the no-vax conflict? This paper exposes observations on this issue based on the analysis of material collected on Telegram, YouTube, Twitter, Facebook, on Telegram groups #@novaxzoneitalia, #@novaxdating, #@politicalleaks, on dedicated YouTube channels as well as of comments that appeared on digital platforms such as *open.online.* The activities of so-called "digital squadrons" were recorded from fall 2020 to early 2022. It is precisely in these contexts that "haters", i.e. people who – often anonymously – act on digital arenas exerting great influence on the group and on public opinion, emerge from the protesting mass. In the analyzed material the following hate speech illocutions were found: discrimination, propaganda and aggression.

Keywords: COVID-19, vaccine conflict, hate speech, haters, verbal aggression, social media communication.

1. Digital spaces in the vaccination conflict

The COVID pandemic kicked off a crisis that transversally affected all European societies, and Italy in particular – the country where the pandemic first hit in Europe in 2019. The decline in trust in institutions, which were considered incapable of dealing with the pandemic (Bucchi, 2021; Campo et al., 2021, 39f.), culminated in Italy with the introduction of compulsory vaccinations in the summer of 2021, stirring up a veritable "vaccination conflict". Numerous protest groups emerged, whose radicalised forms found expression in some cases in violent language that was particularly evident in the media. Among them were so-called "squadrons" of digital warriors[2], i.e. social media groups numbering a few

Silvia Bonacchi, University of Warsaw, ORCID: 0000-0003-3914-1233.

1 The same theme was addressed by me in Bonacchi, 2023.

2 See: https://www.open.online/2020/05/19/coronavirus-e-complottisti-ecco-chi-sono-gli-squadristi-digitali-che-attaccano-le-iene-mentana-lucarelli-barbascura-e-open/, 19 May 2020 (28 June 2024).

hundred members that quickly consolidated into global groups with a variety of names: *no mask*, *no vax*, *free vax*, to name but a few. This "digital squadronism" had a specific programme of action, whose aim was to unmask the alleged "lying and abominable hoax" (14)[3] perpetrated by a supposed vaccine dictatorship, fed by the interests of "Big Pharma", i. e. huge pharmaceutical multinationals.

In this protest movement, we see a renewal of the classic ideological language of hatred that has been typical of dark periods in European history, only this time updated to match the current situation: the authors of social media posts speak of a "Nazi dictatorship", of a "threat to freedom", of the need to "go to war" in order to "save fundamental rights" (all quotations from our corpus). This is a language aimed at tackling perceived "discrimination", understood in the literal sense as an irreducible, unbridgeable opposition between Self and Other (Us and Them, the Healthy and the Sick, the Vaccinated and the Unvaccinated, the Victims and those Responsible), often fuelled by conspiracy narratives about "secret curtains", fake news and infodemic waves aimed at manipulating the masses (Cinelli et al., 2020; Nielsen et al., 2021, Niehr; Czyżewski in this volume).

In this paper we will try to explore to what extent the authors of the posts can be classified as "haters", using a language that bears traits of hate speech, on the basis of observations of material collected on Telegram, YouTube, Twitter, and Facebook, as well as comments that appeared on digital platforms such as *open.online*[4]. The activities were recorded from autumn 2020 to early 2022. In particular, screenshots of posts published (and very often subsequently deleted) on the Telegram groups *#@novaxzoneitalia, #@novaxdating* and *#@politicalleaks*[5], and on dedicated YouTube channels, were collected. The activities of so-called ViVi 'warriors' on Telegram and the #R2020 group on Twitter were also followed. It is precisely in these groups that "haters" emerge from the mass of protestors, i. e. people who act – often anonymously – in digital arenas, not only exerting great influence on the group in question, but also managing to influence public opinion more generally.

3 The fragments analysed in the collected material are numbered consecutively and cited according to the numbering in brackets.

4 Most posts are documented in: https://www.open.online/2021/08/30/covid-19-no-vax-green-pass-squadrismo-digitale/ (12 February 2024).

5 Cf. https://web.telegram.org/k/#@novaxzoneitalia, https://web.telegram.org/k/#@novaxdating, https://web.telegram.org/k/#@politicaleaks (28 February 2023). Many of these groups have currently (09 March 2023) disappeared, and the materials are no longer accessible except in comments in digital newspapers.

2. Hate speech illocutions

The term "hate speech" defines a communication in social arenas based on verbal and non-verbal elements that not only express and spread hatred[6], but above all that makes hatred (as a strong and irrationalising feeling) the moment in which an otherwise weak group is cemented. The fundamental phenomenon in this process is *discrimination*, through which an irreducible opposition is created between the Self and the Other, between Us and Them, which overrides any confrontation with Diversity. The "Diverse" inevitably becomes the "Other", annulling that dynamic inherent in identity processes through which the Self crystallises and defines itself through confrontation with the Other. The Other is thus in hate speech categorically extraneous, and a visceral rejection of the Other results in a structural intolerance and finally in the desire for the Other's annihilation.

Hate speech acts on various levels: on a habitus level it results in hostile attitudes based on bias: on a cognitive level it fosters prejudice: on a behavioural level it fosters discrimination: on an emotional level it induces fear towards an individual or a group of individuals who share an ethnicity, a sexual orientation or a religious faith, a disability, another social or cultural affiliation, or in any case anything that makes them Other.[7] Thus, it is not so much that hate language *expresses hate*, but that it *creates* hate through shared discursive practices (cf. Bonacchi, 2019a, 441; Bonacchi, 2020b, 42). To become the cement of the group[8] hate needs a target, and this target is precisely Diversity. Hatred blocks reason, which seeks to understand and integrate Diversity, fuelling intolerance and violence. In the vaccination conflict, the Others are those who (do not) vaccinate.

Hate speech has a performative character in that it proposes to be translated into action, often resulting in violence. In the vaccine conflict, hate speech is often trivially violent and knows all the tones of confrontation: it starts with attempts at persuasion, moves on to the development of conspiracy narratives, and ends with open aggression (insults, threats and physical violence).

On the basis of Rae Langton's (2012) proposal, we have identified the following "hate illocutions" in the analysed material, i.e. linguistic structures in

6 The European Commission against Racism and Intolerance defines hate speech as follows: "Hate speech covers many forms of expressions which advocate, incite, promote or justify hatred, violence and discrimination against a person or group of persons for a variety of reasons": https://www.coe.int/en/web/european-commission-against-racism-and-intolerance/hate-speech-and-violence/ (28 June 2024).

7 We refer here to the "pyramid of hatred" model developed by the Shoah Foundation (for an extensive discussion see Falloppa 2020: 26): https://www.adl.org/resources/tools-and-strategies/pyramid-hate-student-edition (28 February 2023).

8 Hate speech fuels group cohesion through mechanisms such as mimetic violence and scapegoating (Bonacchi, 2020a; 2019b).

which utterances (verbal utterances and in general iconic and aural messages) convey intended actions:

AGGRESSION, i. e. aggressive (performative, commissive and directive) *acts* such as *persecuting, humiliating, offending, threatening the victim*. These are acts aimed at discrediting or intimidating the victim, denying him/her agentivity (cf. Bonacchi, 2017, 16f.; Bonacchi, 2019a, 440f.).

> Calenda fuck off! Man of <image of excrement>!
> (original Italian: Calenda vaffanculo! Uomo di <immagine di escrementi>!, 18)

> You have to crack heads, you have to crack ankles, you have to crack kneecaps [...]
> (original Italian: Bisogna spaccare teste, bisogna spaccare caviglie, bisogna spaccare rotule [...], 16)

DISCRIMINATION (Us vs. Others) and SUBORDINATION (Us superior to Others):

> Let's protect **our** children! [bolding: SB]
> (original Italian: Proteggiamo i nostri bambini!, 10)

> The blackboard of **good** and **bad** [bolding: SB]
> (original Italian: La lavagna dei buoni e cattivi, 21)

> **You** kill **us** with vaccines, **you** will pay! [bolding: SB]
> (original Italian: Ci uccidete con i vaccini, la pagherete!, 1)

> If **you** don't vaccinate, **I** sincerely hope **you** are disbarred! [bolding: SB] (7)
> (original Italian: Se lei non si vaccina io spero vivamente che lei venga radiato!, 17)

PROPAGANDA[9], i. e. acts in which there is a deliberate and systematic attempt to shape perceptions, manipulate cognition and direct behaviour. Through propaganda, the Ideology – whatever it may be – speaks and the concrete enunciator is depersonalised in favour of an action programme. Propaganda is characterised by language featuring dogmatism, apodicticity, generalisations, programmatic directives, disinformation and manipulation of states of affairs (Udupa et al., 2020, 4f.). Within propaganda, narratives are often developed on the basis of conspiracy theories.

> Freedom against vaccination dictatorship!
> (original Italian: Libertà contro la dittatura vaccinale!, (11)

> Everywhere struggle, everywhere truth, everywhere Vi_Vi
> (original Italian: Ovunque lotta, ovunque verità, ovunque Vi_Vi (12)

> We Vivi [the living persons] will never stop fighting
> (original Italian: Noi Vivi non smetteremo mai di lottare, image 8)

9 See Felling et al., 2019, 12; Baldauf et al., 2015.

In war the one who hits the hardest wins!
(original Italian: In guerra chi mena di più vince!, (20)

[inscriptions on a swastika tattooed on the forehead of public figures graphically reworked:] dictatorship, lies/perbenism[10], lockdown/recession, epidemic/fear
(original Italian: dittatura (5), menzogna/perbenismo (3), lockdown/recessione (4), epidemia/paura (5)

Vaccines kill (9)
(original Italian: I vaccini uccidono, (9)

Many utterances with a complex illocutionary structure were observed, e.g. featuring DISCRIMINATION and AGGRESSION (a threat):

Anyone of **you who** has a business in Italy and illegally dares to **ghettoise anyone who is** [...] will **be targeted, so much shit will be thrown at them that** [...] they **will have to close** [...]! So watch out! [bolding: SB]
(original Italian: Chiunque di voi ha un'attività in Italia e si permette illegalmente di ghettizzare chiunque sia [...] sarà preso di mira, gli verrà rivolta addosso tanta di quella merda che [...] dovrà chiudere [...]! Quindi occhio!, 17)

Or AGGRESSION and PROPAGANDA:

I am a Nazi and I want to impose the Nazi dictatorship (6)
(original Italian: sono un nazista e voglio imporre la dittatura nazi-sanitaria, 6)

In the following, we will try to show the performative character of these illocutions in the collected linguistic material.

3. *Digital squads against the #Nazi_dictatorship*: arenas, agendas, haters and the hated

The vaccination campaign in Europe started at the end of December 2020 with the gradual approval by the European Medicines Agency (EMA) of Pfizer-BioNTech, Moderna, Oxford-Astra Zeneca, Sanofi and Johnson & Johnson vaccines. On 1 July 2021, compulsory vaccination and the *green pass* were introduced in Italy. From spring 2021 onwards, protests started all over Europe. The preferred arenas were the mass media, urban spaces (squares, streets, vaccination hubs) and digital platforms. Above all, social media become a space of aggregation and conflict during the pandemic.[11] Street fighting, demonstrations, and

10 The Italian word "perbenismo", derived from "perbene" (una persona perbene: a decent, respectable person), is in Italian negative and can be translated into English as "pretended respectability".
11 For the principle of *doing aggressive*, see Marx (2017).

marches all developed their maximum effect by becoming viral material, when pictures and short videos were shared in the media.

Particularly active in the analysed groups are so-called "haters". These are individuals and groups with suggestive names (Greg, Zoth, ViVi #R2020) who manage to influence hundreds, and in some cases thousands, of followers. The "haters" play a constitutive role in the process of collective identity formation not only by cementing the group, but also by assigning (or, rather, bullying) or denying a "discursive" role to the victim, i. e. the 'hated'. By subtracting them the role of interlocutors able to negotiate their role, the hated objects are confined to the role of being persons outside the interlocutive relationship. It is a denial of the visibility and agentivity of the interlocutor: there is no discussion with the victim, the victim's role is "inflicted". This is why, in our collected material, targets can be depersonalised, multiplied, and reworked into memes.

The activity of these groups is not so much anonymous as collective. In some cases it is not possible to identify an author of individual messages or memes, while in other cases the author is not important. What is important is that these utterances exist as they are viralised in a process of reduplication, sharing and variation. The utterances thus become an integral part of *shitstorms* against defined targets, in some cases taking on the character of mimetic violence in a digitally consumed collective ritual (cf. Bonacchi, 2020, 143–144). The targets, i. e. the people stigmatised, persecuted and deprived of agentivity – the "hated" – are, this time, not any particular ethnic or social groups, sexual or religious minorities, classically the target of hate speech, but rather those who (do not) vaccinate or who campaign for or against compulsory vaccination (politicians, journalists, doctors), or people who (do not) take the measures envisaged by the authorities against the pandemic (e. g. restaurateurs).

A favoured target in the vaccination conflict are health institutions and doctors – at least according to one plan to eradicate the so-called "iatrodemia" ("iatrodemics", a neologism coined by Nucci & Scaglioni, 2022), i. e. the epidemic of doctors on television propagating "lies", considered a dangerous social pathology.[12] Examples are countless. Among others, Matteo Bassetti, director of the San Martino Polyclinic Hospital in Genoa, appointed spokesman for the Italian Scientists Association, ended up in the eye of the storm. He was chased and threatened by an anti-vaxxer in front of his home with the words:

12 In the vaccination phase of the Covid pandemic, there was a process of spectacularization of science and scientists (primarily doctors, virologists, and biologists), whose unprecedented media exposure was perceived by many as propaganda.

(1) You kill us with vaccines, you will pay![13]
(Original Italian: Ci uccidete con i vaccini, la pagherete!, 1)

A photo of Matteo Bassetti taken from an official website[14] appeared in the digital media[15] after being subjected to graphic reworking programmes. The graphically reworked Bassetti has a swastika on his forehead and speaks through a speech bubble. The image went viral and appeared on social media, including on sites frequented by ViVi groups, on Greg's channel, and on Twitter[16]:

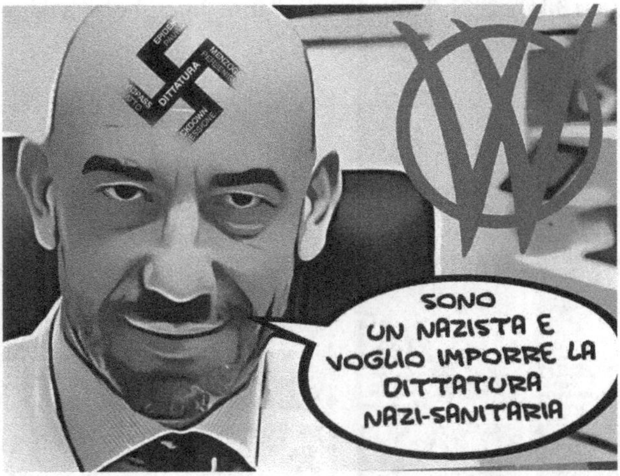

Fig. 1: Graphic reworking of a photo of Matteo Bassetti.

The image is "signed" with a red W inscribed inside a circle, the trademark of the ViVi group. It has no declared author, but by the end of February 2021 at the latest, it started to circulate virally on the web. The reworked photo thus became the starting point for images that developed into narratives. In the graphic reworking, Bassetti wears a swastika on his forehead, in which one can read key words that recur in conspiracy narratives:

(2) dictatorship
(3) lies/"perbenismo"
(4) lockdown/recession
(5) epidemic/fear

13 See https://www.open.online/2021/08/30/covid-19-bassetti-inseguito-no-vax/ (28 February 2023); https://www.open.online/2021/08/31/covid-19-bassetti-inseguito-minacciato-denunce/ (28 February 2023).

14 See https://bsac.org.uk/speakers/matteo-bassetti/ (28 June 2024).

15 See Including Genova24.it, https://www.genova24.it/2022/07/covid-bassetti-sulla-quarta-dose-agli-over60-sara-un-fallimento-annunciato-310329/?amp&amp_js_v=0.1&usqp=mq331AQKKAFQArABIIACAw== (28 June 2024).

16 See https://twitter.com/rossellacucche1 (28 June 2024).

Through the speech bubble, Bassetti in the revised image states:

> I am a Nazi and want to impose a Nazisanitarian dictatorship
> (Original Italian: sono un nazista e voglio imporre la dittatura nazi-sanitaria, 6)

which became a viral statement imposed on targets which also recurred in other reworkings, such as those against TV presenter Bruno Vespa in a memetic composition that appeared on Facebook on the InfoVax group[17]. In the group, which boasts 539 members, graphic reworkings of public figures calling themselves "Nazis" appeared on 3 July 2021. These are similar to "mugshots", with a serial development using a graphic matrix:

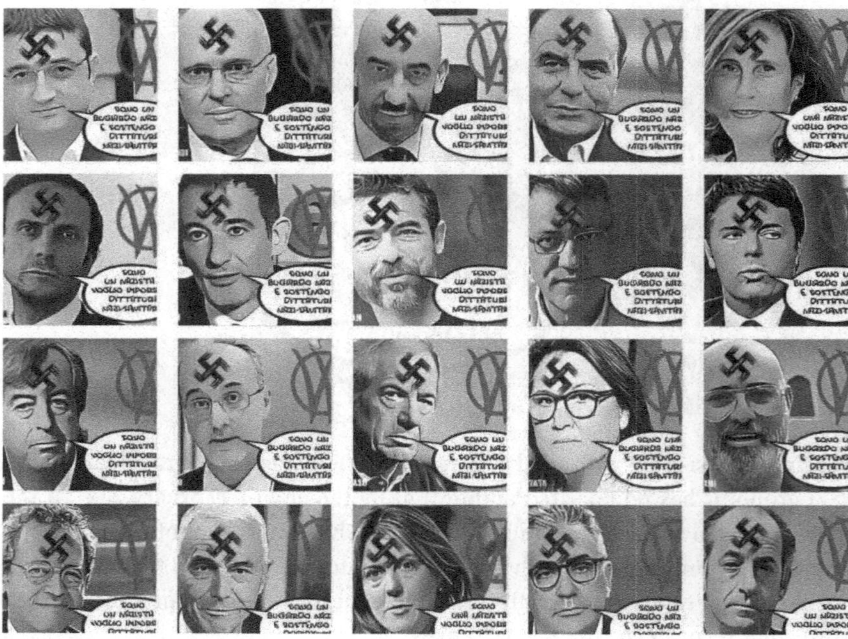

Fig. 2: The photos that appeared on the Infovax group page.

In this memetic composition, the message is repeated as if on multiple mirrors. Among the memes are not only doctors, such as Matteo Bassetti, Ilaria Capua, Roberto Burioni, Giorgio Palù, Pier Luigi Lopalco, Lorenzo Pregliasco and Walter Ricciardi, but also journalists such as Bruno Vespa, Pietro Senaldi, Lucia Annunziata and Enrico Mentana, as well as such politicians as Stefano Bonaccini, Matteo Renzi, Massimiliano Fedriga and Luca Zaia. The memetic composition soon disappeared from the internet due to protests, but individual photos continue to litter the web. The statement (6): "I am a Nazi and I want to impose a Nazi

17 See https://www.facebook.com/groups/infovax (28 June 2024).

dictatorship" is a reference to Bruno Vespa's interruption of doctor Mariano Amici's speech expounding reservations about anticovid vaccination during Rai1's late-night programme *Porta a Porta* (31 March 2021). Bruno Vespa, after an animated exchange of jokes, had intervened decisively, preventing Amici from further laying out his reasons, stating:

> If you do not vaccinate, I sincerely hope you are struck off!
> (Original Italian: Se lei non si vaccina io spero vivamente che lei venga radiato!, 7)

The journalist's intervention was immediately condemned as an act of bullying and an assault on freedom of opinion and televised humiliation[18].

Being branded with the Nazi swastika has also affected personalities such as the politician Andrea Riccardi[19], who via the speech bubble declares, like Bassetti: "I am a Nazi and I want to impose a Nazi-sanitary dictatorship".

An accompanying post reads in capital letters:

> RICCARDI, WHO WAS BURNT AND PISSED OFF. TABLED A MOTION IN THE REGIONAL COUNCIL. THE PATHETIC BUFFOONS ARE VERY CONCERNED ABOUT THE PSYCHOLOGICAL PRESSURE EXERTED BY A CERTAIN TYPE OF STRUGGLE!
> (original Italian: (8) RICCARDI, CHE ERA RIMASTO SCOTTATO E INCAZZATO. HA PRESENTATO UNA MOZIONE IN CONSIGLIO REGIONALE. I NAZISTI PATETICI BUFFONI SONO MOLTO PREOCCUPATI DALLA PRESSIONE PSICOLOGICA ESERCITATA DA UN CERTO TIPO DI LOTTA!, 8)

This is a message identifying the target audience of politicians, who are members of the regional council ("pathetic buffoons"), while also vindicating the actions of the ViVi group, to which the red W, inscribed in a circle, refers. The ViVi (also acronymised as Vi_Vi and V_V) define themselves as "digital warriors" whose aim is to carry out "online raids" against supporters of the vaccination campaign.[20] This is a group that operates via specially created Telegram groups in which conspiracy content[21] is disseminated and in which disruptive acts are shared via pictures or screenshots of what has been vandalised. Members of the group have been invited to carry out protests, such as placing banners or stickers

18 See https://100giornidaleoni.it/tv/mariano-amici-censurato-ed-umiliato-in-diretta-da-bruno-vespa-il-video/ (28 June 2024).

19 Politician Matteo Riccardi in a graphic reworking posted on Telegram (the photo has been removed but is still documented on open.online: https://www.open.online/2021/08/30/covid-19-no-vax-green-pass-squadrismo-digitale/ (28 June 2024).

20 See https://brescia.corriere.it/notizie/cronaca/23_gennaio_29/riunioni-provincia-novax-guerrieri-vivi-nuove-denunce-a1725ee8-9f5c-11ed-a35f-cb762b703658.shtml (28 February 2023).

21 According to an article in the French newspaper *Front Populaire*, this is a group of users who organise themselves on the web to attack anyone who promotes vaccination policy, see https://frontpopulaire.fr/societe/contents/raids-en-ligne-harcelement-quand-une-poignee-dextremistes-anti-vax-affolent_co599161 (28 February 2023).

depicting the group's symbol on institutional premises, in a sort of competition that once even included a bitcoin prize to be awarded to the creator of the most striking act.[22]

From an iconographic point of view, the ViVi symbol is the result of an eclectic convergence of many elements of popular culture 2.0. According to Le Monde, *ViVi* refers to the present indicative or imperative of the verb "to live".[23] The symbol could also refer to the alliterative modern Latin maxim "Vi veri universum vivus vici", i.e.: "By the power of truth, by living, I have conquered the universe", made famous by Alan Moore's graphic novel, illustrated by David Lloyd, entitled *V for Vendetta* (1982–1985), later adapted into a TV series in the 1990s and a film in 2005, in which the phrase is attributed to a generic John Faust. V, in the film, is a revolutionary anarchist who wears a Guy Fawkes mask representing the English Catholic conspirator who took part in the Gunpowder Plot against James I of England in 1605. Just as V turns against the Christian-fascist dictatorship by re-enacting Fawkes' mission, the same conspiratorial mission is re-appropriated by the digital warriors ViVi.

The group publicises acts of vandalism on Telegram, such as one against the Apulian vaccination centre in Cervia and against the then health councillor Pier Luigi Lopalco.

In the post containing the photo of the vaccination hub, we see that, at the entrance to the health facility, a red W symbol inscribed in a circle and a statement have been spray-painted in red paint:

Vaccines kill
(Original Italian: I vaccini uccidono, 9)

To the left we read the declaration:

(10) We protect our children
(Original Italian: Proteggiamo i nostril bambini, 10)

which is a recurring slogan in the European anti-vax campaign, which positions itself as a champion of childhood (another example was demonstrations in Catania on 23 October 2021, in which the demonstrators marched while chanting the slogan: "Hands off the children").

---

22 See https://www.ilsole24ore.com/art/no-vax-fermati-e-denunciati-due-promotori-gruppo-guerriere-vivi-trovate-armi-le-perquisizioni-AEOb1GcC?refresh_ce=1 (28 March 2023). During the last months of 2021, the group became particularly active; as of the beginning of 2023 it seems to have been disbanded.

23 Cf.: https://www.lemonde.fr/pixels/article/2022/01/19/harcelement-en-ligne-arrestations-simultanees-au-sein-d-un-groupe-d-antivax-auteur-de-raids-numeriques-massifs_6110133_4408996.html (28 June 2024) Vi_Vi was also the name of an Italian moped company, founded in the 1950s, which started out as the motorbike division of Viberti.

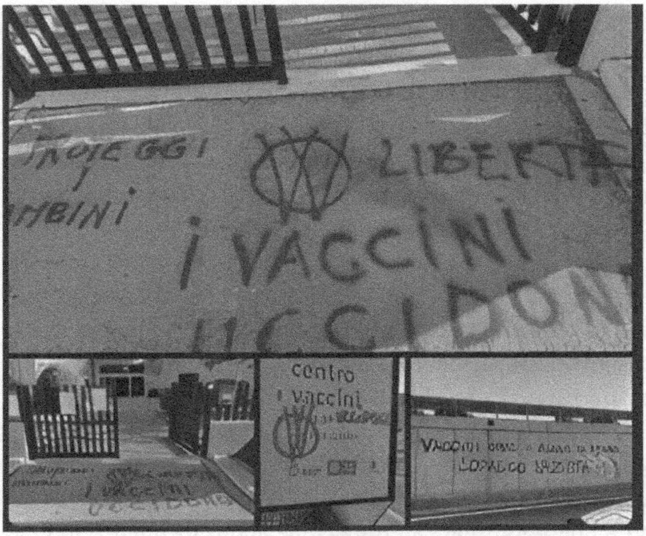

Fig. 3: Detail of the spray-painted graffiti left during the assault on the Cervia vaccination centre.

On the tarmac, not far away, next to the gate we read:

> Freedom against vaccination dictatorship!
> (Original Italian: Libertà contro la dittatura vaccinale!, 11)
>
> Everywhere struggle, everywhere truth, everywhere Vi_Vi
> (Original Italian: Ovunque lotta, ovunque verità, ovunque Vi_Vi, 12)

The ViVi's activities extend to various anti-vaccine "civil distraction" acts. In a 29 July 2021 post on Telegram[24], the ViVi present a plan to sabotage the vaccination campaign by booking appointments they have no intention of keeping, effectively preventing people from getting the vaccine by making them wait until the next round. The post contains actual instructions for followers of the group:

> Book your vaccination appointment for September. If you can, don't do it online. If you cannot then online is ok! If you call and are asked "Why not now?" say that you do not want to ruin your holiday because of possible side effects. And then in September, on the very day of the appointment, you will call to cancel and postpone it. Or you will not show up. The strongest action is to postpone.
> (Original Italian: Prenotate per settembre l'appuntamento con la vaccinazione. Se riuscite non fatelo online. Se non riuscite allora ok online! Se chiamate e vi chiedono "Perché non subito?" dite che non vi volete rovinare le ferie per possibili effetti collaterali. E poi a settembre, il giorno stesso di tale appuntamento, chiamerete per disdire

24 The photo has been removed but is still documented on open.online: https://www.open.online/2021/08/30/covid-19-no-vax-green-pass-squadrismo-digitale/ (28 June 2024).

e rimandare l'appuntamento stesso. Oppure non vi presenterete. L'azione più forte è rimandare, 13)

Another hate-monger railing against supporters of compulsory vaccination was Twitter (@Zoth2021) and Telegram user Zoth[25], currently suspended from both services. In the image[26] published on Telegram by #R2020, a group that defines itself as a "coordination, a democratic, open and inclusive container that brings together all those who fight to reaffirm their rights to freedom, dignity and self-determination", we have the profile of Davide Barillari, a councillor from the Lazio region expelled from the 5 Star Movement for having opened a self-styled counter-information site called "Covid Salute Regione Lazio" and close to the anti-vax movement. In the background, one can make out the cover of Orwell's book. *1984* This juxtaposition of Orwell's *1984* and the new COVID 2019 implicitly re-proposes narratives typical of conspiracy theories: Covid as a multinational conspiracy to overthrow our democratic societies, our fundamental freedoms being threatened by an impersonal fascist regime that permeates the whole of society, and a liberation that can only come about through a spontaneous movement of (now digital) warriors.

Even restaurateurs who reminded customers of the mask requirement and demanded green passes from customers became targets of anti-vax groups. In a post published on Telegram,[27] these measures against the containment of the virus are called a

lying and abominable hoax
(Original Italian: mistificazione bugiarda e abominevole, 14)

Restaurateurs have been overwhelmed by waves of loathing in posts and videos posted on Telegram and YouTube, with exhortations to other group members to "super-share" (Original Italian: Supercondividete!, 15).

These are not only negative comments, but also actions designed to discourage the containment of the virus and the spread of any content undesirable to the anti-vax and conspiracy narratives in general. The waves of hostility often became digital lynch mobs, *shitstorms.* One of the most active groups has been that formed by the Italian YouTuber Gian Luca Gregis ("Greg"), whose activities began in February 2020 with denialist news reports on Covid 19 and culminated

25 The nickname recalls Zoth the Corruptor, a character from the video game World of Warkraft.

26 The photo has been removed but is still documented on open.online: https://www.open.online/2021/08/30/covid-19-no-vax-green-pass-squadrismo-digitale/ (28 June 2024).

27 The photo has been removed but is still documented on open.online: https://www.open.online/2021/08/30/covid-19-no-vax-green-pass-squadrismo-digitale/ (28 June 2024).

in October of the same year[28] with an incitement to his followers (the "gregari") to commit violence against, and murder of, politicians, police officers and journalists. In a video commenting on protest in Naples on 24 October 2020 against Covid regulations, Greg urged his followers to be openly aggressive:

> You have to crack heads, you have to crack ankles, you have to crack kneecaps, I tell you. […] You have to break joints, you have to break elbows, you have to break knees, and when you break people's joints, I assure you they think differently[29]
> (Original Italian: Bisogna spaccare teste, bisogna spaccare caviglie, bisogna spaccare rotule, ve lo dico io. […] Bisogna spaccare le giunture, i gomiti, le ginocchia, allora quando tu alla gente gli spacchi le giunture vi assicuro che ragiona diversamente[30], 16)

In a post[31] accompanying a video published on 28 July 2021 on his own Telegram channel, Radio Greg Original – Free Daily News (with over 17,000 subscribers), Greg announced to his "wingmen" the creation of a public list where all businesses that applied for a green pass would be listed:

> Any of you who has a business in Italy and illegally allows himself to ghettoise whoever it is, as I said, will be targeted, so much shit will be thrown at him that, at the very least, if it goes well he will have lost 50 per cent of his clientele, if it goes badly he will have to close down and many businesses will be shut down! So watch out!
> (Original Italian: Chiunque di voi ha un'attività in Italia e si permette illegalmente di ghettizzare chiunque sia, come ho detto, sarà preso di mira, gli verrà rivolta addosso tanta di quella merda che come minimo, come minimo, se gli va bene ha perso il 50% della clientela, se gli va male dovrà chiudere e molte attività verranno chiuse! Quindi occhio!, 17)

On the same channel, one finds posts insulting a politician called Carlo Calenda who had stated on Twitter that "the rejection of vaccines […] is the rejection of modernity":

> Fuck you Calenda man of <three images of excrement>.
> (Original Italian: Ma vaffanculo Calenda uomo di <tre immagini di escrementi>, 18)

28 During the protest in Naples in October 2020, YouTuber Gregis incites Italians to kill police officers, journalists and politicians, see https://www.open.online/2020/10/24/rivolta-a-napoli-lo-youtuber-gregis-incita-gli-italiani-a-uccidere-poliziotti-giornalisti-e-politici/ (28 June 2024).

29 See https://www.dagospia.com/rubrica-29/cronache/immunita-gregis-delirio-youtuber-gian-luca-gregis-che-250894.htm (28 June 2024).

30 Cfr. https://www.dagospia.com/rubrica-29/cronache/immunita-gregis-delirio-youtuber-gian-luca-gregis-che-250894.htm (28 June 2024).

31 See https://www.open.online/2021/08/30/covid-19-no-vax-green-pass-squadrismo-digitale/ (28 June 2024).

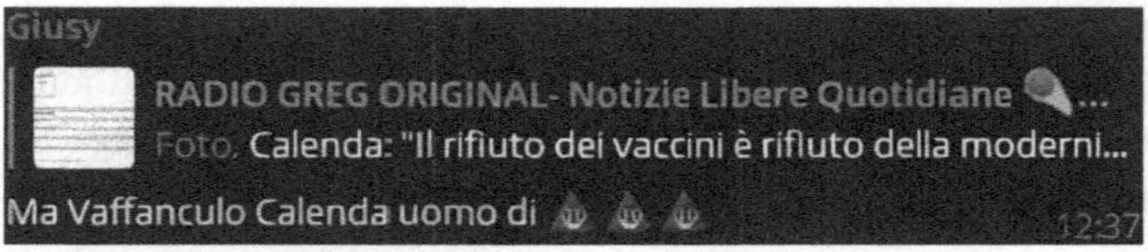

Fig. 4: Comment on Calend's statement.

Greg's threats do not spare his own "wingmen":

> I warn all those who follow me to get to work! If you have activities, do not allow yourselves to do such an action, do not allow yourselves because you will be persecuted! Do not allow yourselves to ghettoise anyone, whoever they are! Not even animals although you are worse than animals, that is! So, don't you dare!
> (Original Italian: Io avviso tutti quelli che mi seguono di darsi da fare! Se avete delle attività non vi permettete di fare un'azione del genere, non vi permettete perché verrete perseguitati! Non vi permettete di ghettizzare chiunque, chiunque sia! Neanche gli animali sebbene voi siete peggio degli animali, ecco! Quindi, non permettetevi!, 19)

And again:

> We are at war, and if we are at war, remember, everything counts! You don't take prisoners in war, you don't discuss morals, ethics, fairness any more, in war whoever hits the hardest wins! Let's see who wins!
> (Original Italian: Siamo in guerra, e se siamo in guerra, ricordatevi, tutto vale! Non si fanno prigionieri in guerra, non si discute più di morale, etica, correttezza, in guerra chi mena di più vince! Vediamo chi vince!, 20)

On the same Telegram group, Radio Greg Chat, user Filo invokes:

> The blackboard of good and bad guys
> (Original Italian: La lavagna dei buoni e cattivi, 21)

followed by Alexander C who believes there is a need to:

> Organise punitive squads.
> (Original Italian: organizzare squadriglie punitive, 22)

4. Conclusion: the anti-vax movement as an expression of popular culture 2.0

At the time of writing it seems that the COVID emergency is over, and with it also the tension related to compulsory vaccination, but other social tensions are looming in Italy and in other Western countries in 2024. In our analysis we have tried to show recurring illocutionary structures in the messages on the digital spaces of the anti-vax protest: aggression in the whole wide range of its variations (offensive comments, threats, exhortations to violence), discrimination (Us and

Them), and what we have called "propaganda", i. e. utterances aimed at shaping perceptions, manipulating cognitions and directing behaviour. Underlying this are forms of denialist conspiracy that feed various types of narratives based on the use of slogans of struggle against lies (especially capitalist ones) and a shadowy conspiracy.

Our observations are limited to a case study. However, we can state, with all the limitations mentioned above, that the groups analysed appear to be deeply rooted in the media and pop-culture, which we have termed "pop-culture 2.0". The utterances and images of hate cease to be individual and are virally reduplicated, shared, reworked, becoming memes, graphic novels and comics. Those hated are depersonalised, reproduced, serialised. Pop-culture 2.0 is not elitist, it is egalitarian, collective, and any content can be appropriated. The starting point for this serialisation process is that content matter is accessible via an average school education, betrayed by references to school set texts and mainstream films. This is a politically indifferent appropriation of the language of traditional hatred, and made possible perhaps thanks to a disturbance in what Vansina (1985, 23–24), in his famous study, called the mechanisms of the *floating gap*, i. e. the detachment from history that allows the formation of a collective memory. In the concrete case of a "Nazi dictatorship", everything can become "Nazism" and "dictatorship" because these concepts are now empty. Which implications will this floating gap bear for our societies of the future?

Works cited

Baldauf, J., Banaszczuk, Y., Koreng, A., Schramm, J. & Stefanowitsch, A. (2015). *"Geh sterben!" Umgang mit Hate Speech und Kommentaren im Internet.* Berlin: Amadeu Antonio Stiftung.

Bonacchi, S. (2017). Sprachliche Aggression beschreiben, verstehen und erklären. Theorie und Methodologie einer sprachbezogenen Aggressionsforschung. In S. Bonacchi (ed.), *Verbale Aggression: Multidisziplinäre Zugänge zur verletzenden Macht der Sprache* (pp. 3–31). Berlin, Munich, Boston: de Gruyter.

Bonacchi, S. (2019a). Verbale Aggression. In F. Liedtke & A. Tuchen (eds.), *Pragmatik-Handbuch* (pp. 439–447). Stuttgart: Springer/Metzler.

Bonacchi, S. (2019b). Perchè le parole fanno male? Considerazioni pragmalinguistiche sull'uso offensivo del linguaggio. In R. Barcellona & T. Sardella (eds.), *Violenza delle parole e parole della violenza. Percorsi storico-letterari tra linguaggi che fanno male e linguaggi che fanno paura* (pp.49–72). Milano: Mimesis.

Bonacchi, S. (2020a). Ostentantiver Sexismus und mimetische Gewalt: Ist Shitstorming gegen Frauen ein Opferritual? In Ł. Kumięga & J. Szczęk (eds.), *Sprache und Gesellschaft. Theoretische und empirische Kontexte der Linguistik* (pp.131–147). Frankfurt a.M. et al.: Peter Lang.

Bonacchi, S. (2020b). Sprachliche Emotionen und verbale Aggression. *Linguistische Treffen in Wrocław*, 17, I, 39–53.

Bucchi, M. (2021). Per aumentare le vaccinazioni investiamo in fiducia. *Nature Italy* 12 January. https://www.nature.com/articles/d43978-021-00004-x (02 February 2023).

Campo, E., Gobo, G., Galeotti, M. & Parra Saiani, P. (2021). Limiti e fallimenti dei modelli epidemiologici e previsionali nell'epidemia di SARS-COV-2. In A. Favretto, A. Maturo & S. Tomelleri (eds.), *L'impatto Sociale del Covid-19* (pp. 39–48). Milan: Angeli.

Cinelli, M., Quattrociocchi, W., Galeazzi, A., Valensise, C.M., Brugnoli, E., Schmidt, A.L., Zola, P., Zollo, F., & Scala, A. (2020). The COVID-19 social media infodemic. *Scientific Reports* 10, 16598. https://www.nature.com/articles/s41598-020-73510-5 (28 February 2023).

Faloppa, F. (2000). *Lessico e alterità: la formulazione del diverso.* Alessandria: Edizioni dell'Orso.

Faloppa, F. (2020). *#Odio. Manuale di resistenza alla violenza delle parole.* Milano: Utet.

Felling, M., Fritzsche, N., Knabenschuh, S. & Schülke, B. (2019). *Hate Speech. Hass im Netz.* Köln: Arbeitsgemeinschaft Kinder- und Jugendschutz (AJS) NRW e.V.

Kahane, A. (2015). Der Kulturkampf der Gegenwart. In J. Baldauf, Y. Banaszczuk, A. Koreng, J. Schramm & A. Stefanowitsch (eds.), *"Geh Sterben!" Umgang mit Hate Speech und Kommentaren im Internet* (pp. 7–8). Berlin: Amadeo Antonio Stiftung.

Langton, R. (2012). Beyond Belief: Pragmatics in Hate Speech and Pornography. In I. Maitra & M.K. McGowan (eds.), *Speech and Harm: Controversies Over Free Speech.* Oxford: Oxford University Press. https://doi.org/10.1093/acprof:oso/9780199236282.003.0004 (28 March 2023).

Marx, C. (2017). "Doing aggressive 2.0" – Gibt es ein genderspezifisches Aggressionsverhalten in der Social-Media-Kommunikation? In S. Bonacchi (ed.), *Verbale Aggression: Multidisziplinäre Zugänge zur verletzenden Macht der Sprache* (pp. 331–355), Berlin, Boston: de Gruyter.

Nielsen, R. K. & Schulz, A., Fletcher, R. (2021). An ongoing infodemic: how people in eight countries access news and information about coronavirus a year into the pandemic. In *Reuters Institute report.* Oxford: Reuters Institute for the Study of Journalism. https://reutersinstitute.politics.ox.ac.uk/ongoing-infodemic-how-people-eight-countries-access-news-and-information-about-coronavirus-year (28 February 2023).

Nucci, P. & Scaglione, M. (2022). *Iatrodemia. Vizi e virtú dei medici in TV.* Milan: Piemme.

Udupa, S., Gagliardone, I., Deem, A., Csuka, L. (2020). Hate Speech, Information, Disorder, and Conflict. Research Review. Social Science Research Council (SSRC), Brooklyn, New York, USA. https://www.ssrc.org/publications/the-field-of-disinformation-democratic-processes-and-conflict-prevention-a-scan-of-the-literature/ (14 April 2025).

Vansina, J. (1985). *Oral Tradition as History.* Madison: University of Wisconsin Press.

Image sources

Fig. 1: Graphic reworking of photo by Matteo Bassetti. https://www.genova24.it/2021/08/pioggia-di-commenti-no-vax-toti-prepara-le-denunce-ecco-chi-sono-i-molestatori-della-w-rossa-271717/ (28 February 2023).

Fig. 2: The 'mugshots' that appeared on the Infovax group (the photo has been removed but is still documented on open.online. https://www.open.online/2021/08/30/covid-19-no-vax-green-pass-squadrismo-digitale/ (28 February 2023).

Fig. 3: Invitation to sabotage the vaccination booking system (the photo has been removed but is still documented on open.online. https://www.open.online/2021/08/30/covid-19-no-vax-green-pass-squadrismo-digitale/ (28 February 2023).

Fig. 4: Comment on Calenda's statement (the photo has been removed but is still documented on open.online. https://www.open.online/2021/08/30/covid-19-no-vax-green-pass-squadrismo-digitale/ (28 February 2023).

Bionotes

Niccolò Bertuzzi is Assistant Professor in Political Sociology and Political Ecology at the University of Parma (Italy). He is a member of different networks, such as ESH Lab (Environmental Social Humanities Lab, UniPr), POLLEN (Political Ecology Network), POE (Politics-Ontologies-Ecologies). He obtained his PhD in Applied Sociology and Methodology of Social Research at University Milano-Bicocca. Among his main research interests: social movement studies, prefigurative politics, conflicts on science and technology, political ecology.
niccolo.bertuzzi@unipr.it

Silvia Bonacchi is Professor at the Institute of Specialized and Intercultural Communication at the University of Warsaw, Poland, and director of the Department for Intercultural Pragmatics and Multimodal Communication. Her research interests cover pragmalinguistics, intercultural communication studies, multimodal communication, conversational and discourse analysis. Her main research fields are (im)politeness and verbal aggression, digital communication, multilingualism and multiculturalism. Her relevant works for the presented volume are the monographs *(Un)Höflichkeit – Eine kulturologische Analyse Deutsch-Italienisch-Polnisch* (2013), *Verbale Aggression: Multidisziplinäre Zugänge zur verletzenden Macht der Sprache* (ed., 2017), *Vulnerability* (ed. 2024) and several papers dedicated to discourse analysis.
s.bonacchi@uw.edu.pl

Enrico Campo is a research fellow of Sociology at the Department of Philosophy, University of Milan (Italy) where he teaches Sociological theory. His research interests also include sociology of knowledge and the study of the relations among culture, technology and cognition. He is the author of *Attention and its Crisis in Digital Society* (2022), co-editor of *Politics of Curiosities. Alternatives to the Attention Economy* (with Yves Citton, 2024) and *Exploring the Crisis. Theoretical Perspectives and Empirical Investigations* (with Andrea Borghini, 2015).
enrico.campo@unimi.it

Marek Czyżewski is Professor Emeritus at the Institute of Sociology, University of Łódź, Poland. His main interests include: discourse analysis; public and mass communication; public opinion and democracy; hate speech; "governmentality"; intercultural and international communication; social theory (especially interpretive approaches, sociology of knowledge, and Foucault). Editor-in-chief of *Przegląd Socjologiczny*; editor of the series *Biblioteka Dyskursu Publicznego.* Among his publications are: *Öffentliche Kommunikation und Rechtsextremismus* (2005, author), *Discourse of Symbolic Elites. An Attempt at Diagnosis* (2014, in Polish, co-editor and co-author), and *Analysis of Public Discourse. Review of Methods and Approaches* (2017, in Polish, co-editor).
marek.czyzewski2012@gmail.com

Giampietro Gobo is Professor of Science and Technology Studies at the University of Milan. His interests concern the sociology of senses and scientific controversies on health issues. He is currently undertaking ethnographic experiments on the role of senses in teamwork cooperation, and research on the pediatric immunizations and COVID-19 policies. His books include *Doing Ethnography* (2008), *Qualitative Research Practice* (co-edited with C. Seale, J. F. Gubrium and D. Silverman, 2004), *Constructing Survey Data: An Interactional Approach* (with S. Mauceri, 2014), *Merged Methods: A Rationale for Full Integration* (with N. Fielding, G. La Rocca and W. van der Vaar, 2021) and *Science, Technology and Society: An Introduction* (with V. Marcheselli, 2023).
giampietro.gobo@unimi.it

Małgorzata Godlewska is Assistant Professor at the Institute of Applied Linguistics at the University of Gdańsk. Her academic interests oscillate between translation studies, translation didactics, discourse analysis and media studies. Her latest research focuses on multimodality in relation to critical discourse analysis and teaching translation as well as on multilingualism and multiculturalism and their transfer in the process of audiovisual translation. Her most recent publications: Building translation sub-competences of foreign language students in telecollaboration (2023) in H. Lankiewicz (ed.) *Extending research horizons in applied linguistics between interdisciplinarity and methodological diversity*; Multilingual transfer and redundancy in audiovisual translation of Woody Allen's polyglot film genre (2024) in *Translation – Didactics of Translation – Pedagogical Translation* (co-editor with J. Hinc).
malgorzata.godlewska@ug.edu.pl

Łukasz Kumięga is Assistant Professor at the Institute of Applied Linguistics, University of Gdańsk. He is a linguist, discoursologist, interested in relationships between language and social processes. Author of a monograph on street demonstrations of extreme right-wing movements in Germany, *Rechtsextremistischer Straßendiskurs in Deutschland* (2013), co-editor of 10 multi-author monographs from the area of interdisciplinary relationships of linguistics with other humanities and social sciences (e.g. *Analysing Discourse, Analysing Poland. The Case of a Political Interview* (2023), *Pädagogisch-fremdsprachendidaktische Verortungen der Lehrerforschung. Konzepte, Herausforderungen, Perspektiven* (2021), and *Sprache und Gesellschaft. Theoretische und empirische Kontexte der Linguistik* (2020). Currently conducting research at the intersection of language, discourse, education and migration.
Lukasz.Kumiega@ug.edu.pl

Elisa Lello is Assistant Professor in Political Sociology and Methodology of Social and Political Research at the University of Urbino (Italy). Her research interests include: traditional and emerging forms of political engagement; territorial inequalities and neo-populism, with a specific interest in inner/rural areas; and youth civic/political engagement. In recent years, her research has mainly focused on the relationship between science, epistemology and politics: the scientization of politics, technoscientific conflicts, science-related populism. Relevant publications for this volume include the book (edited with Niccolò Bertuzzi) *Dissenso informato* (2022) and several scientific articles analysing the protests related to vaccine hesitancy and the roots of social criticism of science.
elisa.lello@uniurb.it

Thomas Niehr is Professor at the Institute for Linguistics and Communication Studies at RWTH Aachen University, Germany. His research interests include language and politics studies, discourse analysis, and linguistic language criticism. He particularly focuses on argumentation analysis. Relevant works for the presented paper include numerous articles on argumentation analysis and conspiracy theories.
t.niehr@isk.rwth-aachen.de

Luca Serafini is a tenure-track assistant professor in Sociology of Cultural and Communication Processes at the University of Florence (Italy). His research interests cover media studies, sociology of journalism, Science and Technology Studies. His relevant works for the presented volume are: The socio-pragmatic dimension of truth. How knowledge claims refused by science find support in public discourse (2023) in *Rassegna Italiana di Sociologia*; Disentangling Discursive Spaces of Knowledge Refused by Science: An Analysis of the Epistemic

Structures in the Narratives Repertoires on Health During the Covid-19 Pandemic (2024) in *Manufacturing Refused Knowledge in the Age of Epistemic Pluralism.*
luca.serafini@unifi.it

Ingo H. Warnke is Professor and holds the Chair of German Linguistics and Interdisciplinary Linguistics at the University of Bremen. His research focuses on Discourse Analysis, the modern and recent history of German language with a special focus on language in colonial archives and in the field of Contradiction Studies. His most recent works include *Sansibarzone* (2020) together with Anna Storch, *Handbuch Sprache im urbanen Raum* (2022) with Beatrix Busse and *Handbuch Diskurs* (2018).
iwarnke@uni-bremen.de